Cerebral Palsy - Updates

Edited by Pinar Kuru Bektaşoğlu

Published in London, United Kingdom

Cerebral Palsy - Updates
http://dx.doi.org/10.5772/intechopen.102254
Edited by Pinar Kuru Bektaşoğlu

Contributors
Yasser Awaad, Marian Sankombo, Christian Chukwukere Ogoke, Nathaniel Larbi Andah, Shin Ushiro, Shiv Lal Yadav, Raj Kumar, Pinar Kuru Bektaşoğlu

First published in London, United Kingdom, 2023 by IntechOpen
IntechOpen is the global imprint of INTECHOPEN LIMITED, registered in England and Wales, registration number: 11086078, 5 Princes Gate Court, London, SW7 2QJ, United Kingdom

British Library Cataloguing-in-Publication Data
A catalogue record for this book is available from the British Library

Additional hard and PDF copies can be obtained from orders@intechopen.com

Cerebral Palsy - Updates
Edited by Pinar Kuru Bektaşoğlu
p. cm.
Print ISBN 978-1-80356-581-1
Online ISBN 978-1-80356-582-8
eBook (PDF) ISBN 978-1-80356-583-5

For EU product safety concerns:
IN TECH d.o.o., Prolaz Marije Krucifikse Kozulić 3, 51000 Rijeka, Croatia,
info@intechopen.com or visit our website at intechopen.com.

Meet the editor

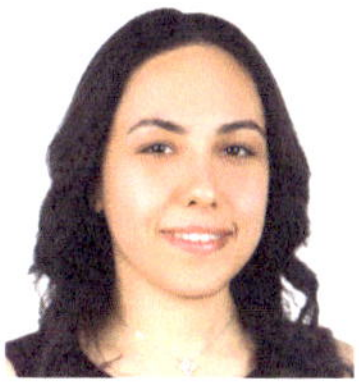

Dr. Kuru Bektaşoğlu graduated from Marmara University School of Medicine, Turkey, in 2014. She completed her neurosurgical residency in 2021 and her Ph.D. in Physiology at Marmara University Institute of Health Sciences, also in 2021. She worked as a research fellow in the Department of Neurological Surgery, at Yeditepe University, Turkey for six months studying white matter fiber dissection. She has given more than seventy presentations at international and national meetings and published forty papers both in peer-reviewed journals. She has also written two books and eight book chapters. She has a keen interest in neurovascular and neurooncological surgeries and translational neuroscience.

Contents

Preface

Cerebral palsy is defined as "a group of permanent disorders of the development of movement and posture, causing activity limitation, that is attributed to non-progressive disturbances that occurred in the developing fetal or infant brain." It is the most common motor disability seen in childhood. Cerebral palsy is caused by abnormal brain development or damage to the developing brain that results in a person's inability to control his or her muscles. The most common structural problem is within the white matter of the brain. It may occur during pregnancy, delivery, the first month of life, or less commonly in early childhood. There are four types of cerebral palsy: spastic, dyskinetic (also includes athetoid, choreoathetosis, and dystonic cerebral palsies), ataxic, and mixed types. The most common of those is the spastic type of cerebral palsy. Although there are treatment alternatives for cerebral palsy, there is still room for improving the medical care of patients with cerebral palsy.

This book includes seven chapters covering etiology and pathophysiology of cerebral palsy, and social impacts of the disease. It also examines current treatment modalities for cerebral palsy.

Pinar Kuru Bektaşoğlu
Sivas Numune Hospital,
Department of Neurosurgery,
Sivas, Turkiye

Section 1

Aetiology and Pathophysiology

Chapter 1

Aetiology and Pathophysiology of Cerebral Palsy

Christian Chukwukere Ogoke

Abstract

The accurate identification of the actual causes (aetiology) of cerebral palsy (CP) and understanding the causal pathways and the neuropathological correlations are critical to the development of both prevention strategies and a holistic classification of CP. The aetiology of CP is multifactorial with diverse and complex causal mechanisms. It has remained a challenge to identify all the non-progressive disturbances and causal pathways in CP despite pivotal contributions from recent advances in neuroimaging. The objectives of this chapter are to discuss the risk factors for CP, elucidate the causal pathways based on current perspectives and explain the pathophysiology of the clinical manifestations of an abnormally developing or damaged motor system. It is expected that at the end of this chapter, the reader should be able to comprehend the challenge in accurately identifying the actual causes of CP and understanding the complex causal pathways and explain the protean clinical features of CP.

Keywords: cerebral palsy, aetiology, risk factor, pathophysiology, multifactorial, causal pathway

1. Introduction

The accurate identification and understanding of the actual causes (aetiology) of cerebral palsy (CP), timing of insults, the causal pathways, mechanisms and "hows" and "whys" (pathophysiology/neuropathological correlations) are critical to the development of both prevention strategies and a holistic or standardized classification of CP [1, 2]. However, it has remained a challenge to identify the non-progressive disturbances or events and causal pathways/processes that led to the damage to the developing motor system in the foetal/infant brain since most of these factors are antenatal in timing [1, 3]. Though there are significant contributions from recent advances in neuroimaging to our understanding of the aetiology and pathology of CP and timing of insults, there are still limitations and these have debarred the emergence of a comprehensive neuropathologic classification of CP [1, 2, 4].

It is obvious that CP is not a single disorder/disease but a group of aetiologically heterogeneous disorders. This implies the aetiology is multifactorial and the causal mechanisms multiple and complex [1, 5]. Thus, various aetiological/risk factors act through multiple pathways to damage the developing motor system resulting in variable phenotypes (clinical subtypes of CP) that have common denominators: abnormal pattern of posture and/or movement and presence of accompanying impairments. Therefore, in simplistic terms, a plethora of factors acting at different times and more commonly in combination interfere with brain development or specifically increase the risk of damage to the developing motor system in the brain (CP).

2. Aetiology/risk factors for cerebral palsy

2.1 Aetiology or risk factors?

The most recent definition of cerebral palsy stipulates that the disorders collectively termed cerebral palsy are attributed to non-progressive disturbances that occurred in the developing foetal or infant brain [6]. The non-progressive disturbances refer to events or processes that within a limited period/duration (static in nature) permanently damage the brain (specifically motor development) or influence the expected patterns of brain maturation [1, 6]. Many different processes or events can result in this damage and so CP is understandably said to be aetiologically heterogeneous (due to multiple aetiologies) and compatible with many aetiologic diagnoses [1, 4]. Indeed, CP on its own is not an aetiologic diagnosis [1]. Furthermore, CP is pathologically heterogeneous since different aetiological factors acting at different stages of development result in different neuropathological substrates even if they lead to the same clinical subtype [4]. For instance, both severe neonatal encephalopathy from perinatal asphyxia and kernicterus from severe unconjugated hyperbilirubinaemia are different aetiological factors for dyskinetic (choreoathetoid/dystonic) CP but they damage different parts of the brain (the ventrolateral nucleus of the thalamus and putamen versus globus pallidus and subthalamic nucleus, respectively) [7, 8].

Direct causal links or relationships are difficult to establish with certainty and explains why the phrase "attributed to" is used in the most recent definition with respect to the causes of CP instead of "are due to" or "caused by" [1, 6]. Therefore, risk factors (correlational) that increase the probability or chances of occurrence of CP are epidemiologically more appropriate than causes. The significance of identification/knowledge of actual causes/risk factors of CP is its implication for prevention. That is, it will help devise prevention strategies for CP.

2.2 Identification of the actual causes of CP: the challenge

The accurate identification of the specific disturbance or specific timing of the event or process that damaged the developing motor system has remained difficult since most (about 75%) of the events occur in the antenatal (prenatal) period [1, 6]. There is also a challenge in designing prospective studies to identify risk factors across populations since only 2–3 per 1000 pregnancies will result in a child with CP [3]. However, neuroimaging has made significant contribution to the understanding of the aetiology and pathology of CP and timing of insults [4 5]. Neuroimaging can be used to identify the neuropathological substrates of the various aetiologic or risk factors of CP, possibly provide information about timing of insults and detect cerebral dysgenesis [2, 4]. Nevertheless, there exists some limitations presently as neuropathologic—aetiological correlations are not yet fully clear and comprehensive [4].

2.3 Causal pathways/mechanisms

Certainly a large number of risk factors are associated with CP and have been identified in numerous earlier studies [9–15] in different parts of the world. These studies have shown that in many cases it is not a single factor but a combination of risk factors (multifactorial) or a cascade of events or disturbances that result in CP [3, 16, 17]. This gave birth to the concept of causal pathways or mechanisms in CP causation and in disorders without a single definitive cause.

According to Stanley et al. [18], a causal pathway refers to a sequence of interdependent events that culminate in disease. This implies that one risk factor leads to another, to another and so on ultimately resulting to the disorder or disease. For instance, prematurity is an important risk factor for CP and can lead to periventricular leukomalacia (white matter injury), poor lung development or respiratory distress at birth, birth asphyxia, increased risk of chronic bilirubin encephalopathy (kernicterus) and so on, ultimately resulting in CP. Nevertheless, prematurity alone is not a sufficient cause for CP since not all children born prematurely have CP. Another example is breech presentation at birth leads to increased risk of cranial trauma or injury and increased risk of CP in places where breech delivery per vaginam is rife.

From the foregoing, it is obvious that the risk factors in a pathway are interconnected and in most cases additively increase the risk of CP. This explains the "two-hit" and "multi-hit" models that consider accumulation of risk factors/insults and a synergistic increase in risk in causation of CP [16, 19]. That is, the brain of a neonate with in-utero exposure to placental inflammation (chorioamnionitis/funisitis/chronic vasculitis) or who had foetal growth restriction ("first-hit") is more vulnerable or conditioned to another injury like sepsis in the neonatal period ("second-hit") ("two-hit" model) while exposure to three or more adverse events/risk factors underlies the "multiple-hit model" of CP causation [16, 19]. Another example of interaction of risk factors is the increased cumulative risk of CP in a child with co-occurrence of early-onset pre-eclampsia, foetal infection/foetal inflammatory response syndrome (FIRS), perinatal asphyxia and neonatal sepsis [19].

One identifiable challenge is that there are so many possible and complex pathways since the risk factors are numerous and each pregnancy presents new possibilities [19]. Some examples of known CP causal pathways are shown in **Figures 1–4** below. The significance of identifying and understanding all these complex causal pathways is in formulating preventive strategies as earlier mentioned. Thus, more research is needed to elucidate the combined effect and specific sequence of multiple risk factors on the occurrence of CP.

2.4 Aetiology of cerebral palsy: historical vs. current perspectives and well-resourced/high income countries (HICs) vs. low & Medium Income countries (LMICs)

Historically, William J. Little and Sigmund Freud made significant contributions to the understanding of the aetiology of CP [20]. In brief, Little first described spastic diplegia (Little's disease) and causally related it to difficult delivery, preterm birth and birth asphyxia—a conception that has survived centuries [5, 20]. However, Freud was the first to state that CP could result solely from antenatal or intrauterine factors (in utero abnormalities of brain development) or combined with birth complications [5, 20]. This assertion which was at variance with that of Little derived from

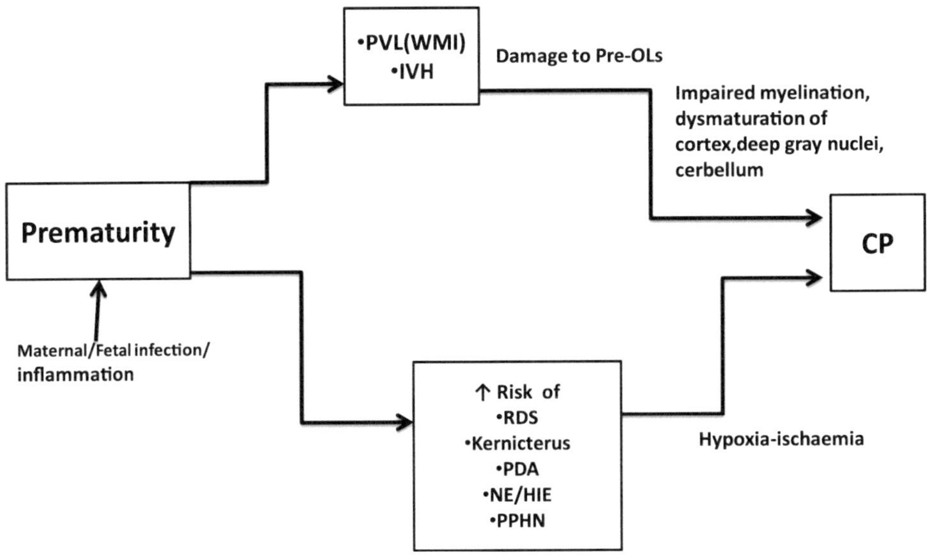

Figure 1.
Casual pathway from prematurity to CP.

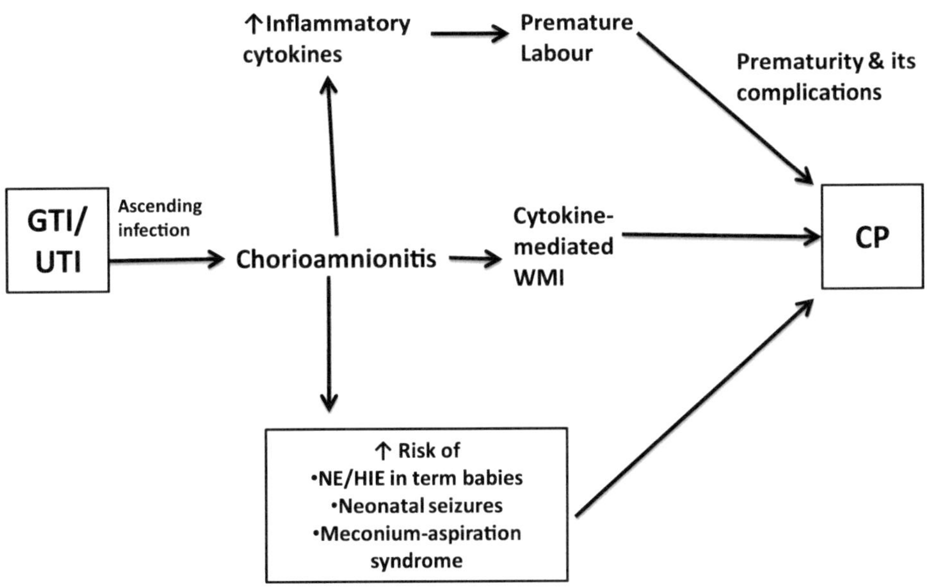

Figure 2.
Causal pathway from maternal genitourinary tract infection to CP.

his observations that children with CP had many other neurological disorders and children with birth asphyxia could be completely normal [5, 20]. Nevertheless, the contribution of the perinatal period to CP causation (Little's view) has also been supported by subsequent research [16]. But this is indeed much less frequent than previously thought.

Current understanding of the aetiology of CP support more of Freud's views since epidemiological studies [9, 10] notably the National Collaborative Perinatal Project [9]

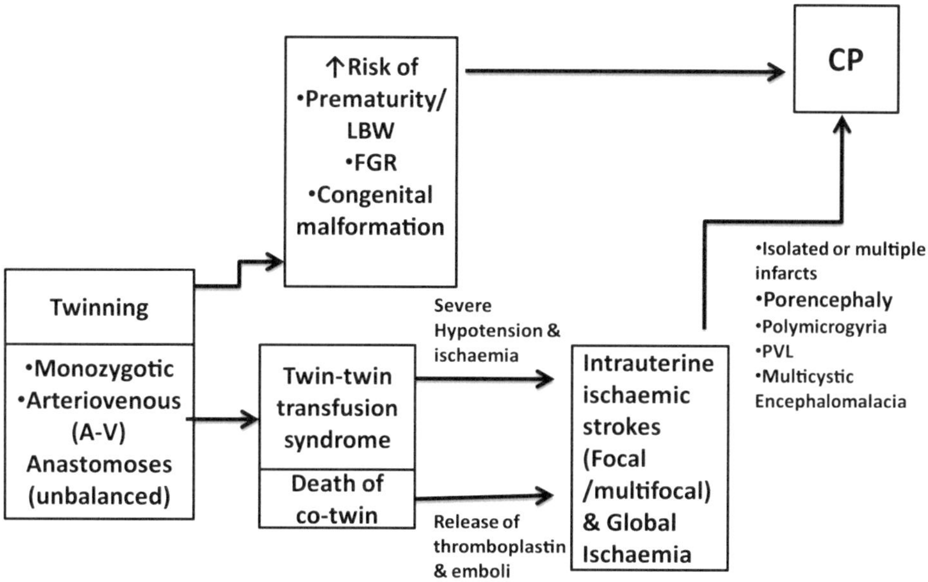

Figure 3.
Casual pathway from twinning to CP.

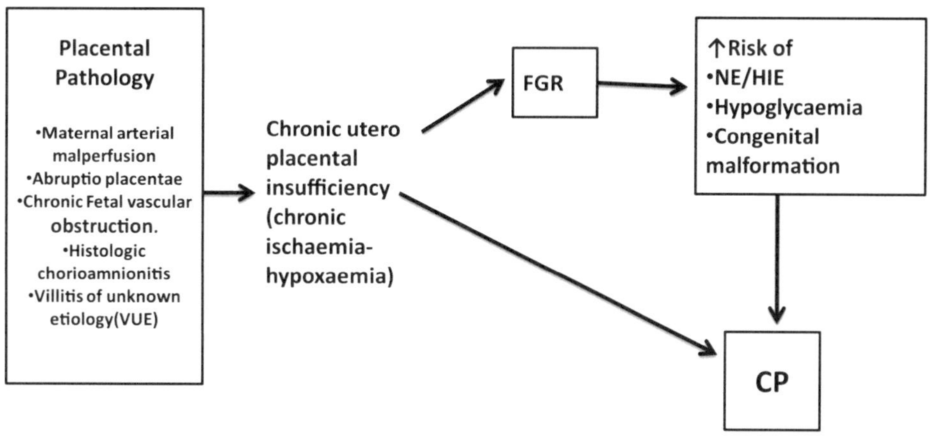

Figure 4.
Casual pathway from placental pathology to CP.

brought to the fore that less than 10 percent of CP were causally related to birth asphyxia but rather most predictors of CP were antenatal factors [10]. Thus, the debate on causation and timing has moved from intrapartum events (birth asphyxia, birth trauma/complications, Little's view) to antenatal factors or antecedents (cerebral dysgenesis, genetics, maternal infection, Freud's view) [4, 9, 10]. Further support for the significant role of antenatal factors or "antecedents" in CP causation is the fact that the reduction in perinatal asphyxia by improved perinatal and obstetric care in well-resourced countries (HICs) of Europe and America did not lower the prevalence of CP [21]. Recent studies involving neuroimaging and inflammatory markers [22–25] which continue to debunk Little's view of birth asphyxia as a major cause of CP abound in literature from developed countries of Europe and America. However, studies from low and middle income countries (LMICs) of Africa continue to implicate preventable perinatal and postnatal aetiological factors in CP (perinatal asphyxia, kernicterus, meningitis, cerebral malaria) [26]. Majority of these studies are of low-quality with simple cross-sectional design and lacking appropriate control groups for proper assessment of risk factors [26]. The studies involving neuroimaging and inflammatory markers are rare in LMICs due to financial constraints, unavailability of equipment and lack of expertise. Therefore, the type and quality of studies on aetiological factors in CP seen in well-resourced countries are needed in developing countries (LMICs) to harmonize the spectrum of aetiological factors and timing of insults in CP worldwide.

As regards the relative contribution of individual risk factors to CP causation, variations also exist between HICs and LMICs. It is well known that in HICs, improved preventive measures, use of guidelines and better management of neonatal jaundice have resulted in a significant reduction of cases of CP attributed to kernicterus [27]. Moreso, prolonged obstructed labour and breech delivery with its attendant increased risk of intracranial haemorrhage/injury are currently rare in HICs owing to the high rates of planned caesarean deliveries [19]. Furthermore, congenital rubella infection and meningitis caused by *Haemophilus influenzae* Type B (HIB) and Neisseria meningitidis have been significantly reduced through effective immunization programmes in HICs while the recent introduction of the malaria vaccine is expected to reduce the relative contribution of cerebral malaria to brain damage in malaria-endemic regions [27]. The reducing incidence and severity of CP associated with prematurity has been reported in some HICs [28]. Further reduction in the prevalence of CP among children with low birth weight is expected with the implementation in many HICs of guidelines recommending administration of magnesium sulphate ($MgSO_4$) for neuroprotection in imminent preterm delivery at <32–34 weeks of gestation (pre-eclampsia and preterm labour) [19, 28].

2.5 Comprehensive list of risk factors for CP

A comprehensive list of risk factors for CP does not exist and a number of cases may be devoid of known risk factors. A plethora of epidemiological studies [3, 9–25] worldwide have been done to ascertain risk factors for CP and have reported countless risk factors for CP categorized as antenatal (prenatal), perinatal (natal) or postnatal (postneonatal) in timing. A meta-analysis [29] of 18 studies in China identified six major risk factors for CP during pregnancy namely: advanced maternal age (≥ 35 years), multiple pregnancy, medicine use in early pregnancy, harmful environment, recurrent vaginal bleeding during pregnancy and pregnancy-induced hypertension (pre-eclampsia). A systematic review [26] of 25 articles identified 10 consistent risk factors (statistically significant in each study) for CP in children born at term in well-resourced countries/HICs namely: placental abnormalities, major and minor birth defects, low birth weight, meconium aspiration, instrumental/emergency caesarean delivery, birth asphyxia, neonatal seizure, respiratory distress syndrome, hypoglycaemia and neonatal infections. Another systematic review of paediatric cerebral palsy in Africa [26] reported that the most common risk factors identified in African cohorts were birth asphyxia, kernicterus and neonatal infections. From the foregoing, it is already clear that there are numerous risk factors for CP with variations in the spectrum of risk factors for preterm and term babies (different gestation ages), HICs and LMICs and strength of associations (some strongly correlated and others weakly associated).

Pre-pregnancy/maternal factors: low socioeconomic status, maternal medical conditions (server maternal iodine deficiency/thyroid disorder, intellectual disability, epilepsy)
Antenatal: prematurity, genetic factors/mutations, congenital malformations/cerebral dysgenesis, placental pathology, infections (TORCH, maternal genitourinary infections), Intrauterine growth restriction (IUGR/FGR/SGA), multiple births, antepartum haemorrhage
Perinatal: perinatal asphyxia/birth complications, neonatal encephalopathy, perinatal stroke, kernicterus
Postnatal (postneonatal): meningitis/encephalitis (including cerebral malaria), kernicterus, traumatic head injuries, shaken baby syndrome, cardiopulmonary arrest (near drowning)

TORCH syndrome refers to transplacental &/parturitional infections with Toxoplasmosis, Others (syphilis, HIV, EBV, Zika, varicella, enterovirus), Rubella, Cytomegalovirus, Herpes simplex. FGR = Foetal Growth restriction. SGA = Small for Gestational Age.

Table 1.
Risk factors for cerebral palsy.

Table 1 shows a list of risk factors for CP but the list is inexhaustive since many cases of CP have unidentifiable aetiological factors. Subsequently, a discussion of some of the risk factors with emphasis on their neuropathological substrates will follow.

3. Neuropathological substrates of some significant risk factors for CP

An awareness of the neuropathology of CP will facilitate comprehension of the clinico-pathological correlates of CP—the phenotypes, clinical features and the accompanying physical, mental or physiological impairments.

3.1 Prematurity and CP

Prematurity plays a relatively greater role in CP causation in HICs (increased survival of preterm babies due to advanced healthcare systems) than in resource-poor countries where the mortality rate of preterm/low birth weight babies remains high [19]. Studies have shown that the prevalence of CP is inversely proportional to gestational age and indeed a meta-analysis reports rates of 111.80 per 1000 live births in infants born <28 weeks and 1.35 per 1000 for children born after 36 weeks [30]. Some factors postulated to contribute to this increased prevalence of CP among children born preterm include: infection/inflammation, organ immaturity, hormone and growth factor deficiency, metabolic factors, environmental factors and pregnancy-related complications [19]. In a word, prematurity increases susceptibility of the foetus to multiple insults or accumulation of risk factors ("multiple hit phenomena") by increased predisposition to infection/inflammation, periventricular leukomalacia (PVL), periventricular-intraventricular haemorrhage, Persistent pulmonary hypertension of the newborn (PPHN), Respiratory Distress Syndrome (RDS), perinatal asphyxia, Patent Ductus Arteriosus (PDA), encephalopathy of prematurity, mechanical ventilation, unconjugated hyperbilirubinaemia and so on (see **Figure 1** above). This may explain why prematurity is a major risk factor for CP.

In prematurity, the neuropathological substrate for CP is a hypoxia-ischaemia-infection-inflammation-glutamate excitotoxic-free radical-cytokine-mediated cerebral white matter injury termed periventricular leukomalacia (PVL) [31]. The selective vulnerability of the periventricular white matter to injury during this gestational period (24–34 weeks GA) relates to factors such as vascular immaturity/arterial end zones in the periventricular region, significantly lower basal blood flow to cerebral white matter, pressure-passive cerebral blood flow, high angiogenesis and high proliferation, maturation and migration of glial cells and premyelinating oligodendrocytes (pre-OLs) [31]. PVL manifests a spectrum of severity with the most severe injury resulting in focal necrotic cysts (cystic PVL) and focal necrotic but non-cystic gliotic scars (appears as punctuate white matter lesions on MRI) while mild injuries result in diffuse white matter gliosis that is non-necrotic and non-cystic termed chronic white matter injury (CWMI) [32]. The latter appears on MRI as diffuse excessive high signal intensity (DEHSI) [32]. Obviously, the more severe lesions of cystic PVL (focal cysts) are correlated more frequently with bilateral spastic CP (spastic diplegia) and also with more severe motor deficits than the less striking diffuse CWMI [32, 33]. Fortunately, owing to mitigation of preterm cerebral injury through improved neonatal intensive care in HICs, cystic PVL is currently rare (<5%) in very preterm infants [31]. This has contributed to some reports of dwindling prevalence of CP associated with prematurity and significantly the occurrence of less severe motor deficits [28, 32]. However, the currently predominant diffuse CWMI in infants born prematurely translates to prominent cognitive disturbance, albeit with minor motor deficits [32].

Ultimately, the result of PVL is delayed/impaired myelination caused by loss or damage to the oligodendrocyte precursors (pre-OLs) in the periventricular region [32]. The higher prevalence of preterm/LBW babies in HICs may partly explain why white matter lesions are the commonest MRI findings in children with CP [28, 32]. It also contributes to spasticity being the most prevalent CP type since more medial PVL damages descending corticospinal (pyramidal) tracts for lower limb control resulting in spastic diplegia (spastic bilateral CP) and with more severe lesions (lateral extension to the centrum semiovale and internal capsule) affect upper limbs and intellectual functions in addition—spastic quadriplegia (spastic bilateral CP) [28, 31, 32]. Thus, in spastic CP, the severity of motor deficit/functional impairment and frequency of accompanying impairments correlate with the severity and extent of brain injury [31, 32].

3.2 Infection, inflammation and CP

There is a consensus in the literature that infections/inflammation via cytokine-mediated injury to the immature brain are causally associated with CP (see **Figure 2**). Infection, inflammation and cytokines play a fundamental role in CP causation through their link with preterm labour (prematurity), placental pathology (chorioamnionitis, funisitis), congenital malformation, FGR, cerebral white matter injury (WMI) and perinatal asphyxia [29, 33–37]. Studies including recent meta-analyses have shown compelling evidence that maternal infections in pregnancy, intra-amniotic infection (chorioamnionitis), evidence of FIRS and neonatal infections are causally associated with CP [25, 29, 35–37]. Both transplacental TORCH infections (Toxoplasmosis, Others [syphilis, Epstein Barr virus, HIV, Zika virus], Rubella, Cytomegalovirus [CMV], Herpes virus), genitourinary infections (bacterial vaginosis, chlamydia, trichomonas, UTI) and neonatal infections (GBS-early onset sepsis, neonatal pneumonia, meningitis) have all been implicated in CP [37]. Many studies [22–25] in the twentieth and twenty-first centuries have suggested that inflammatory phenomena/infections play a more critical role in the aetiology of brain lesions common in CP. Additionally, placental histology should be requested for in babies compromised at birth since chorioamnionitis, funisitis (umbilical cord inflammation) (placental pathology) are evidence of infection predating labour [17].

In the setting of infection/inflammation, one neuropathological substrate for CP is a cytokine-mediated cerebral white matter injury (PVL) in the preterm infant, though minimal evidence exists for such a process in term newborns [37]. Other mechanisms include: brain damage/cerebral dysgenesis by TORCH infections especially CMV, direct cytokine toxicity to premyelinating oligodendrocytes (pre-OLs), hypoxic brain damage by neonatal pneumonia with PPHN, ischaemic cerebral damage from microvascular thrombosis and hypoperfusion in neonatal meningitis et cetera [31, 33, 37].

3.3 Cerebral dysgenesis and CP

Disruption of the development of motor pathways that control movement and posture is the underlying pathogenesis of CP attributed to cerebral malformations. Cerebral dysgenesis has a firm causal link with CP and both cerebral and non-cerebral malformations increase the likelihood of CP [17, 19]. Some brain malformations have genetic causes like LIS1 and doublecortin (DCX), TUBA1A mutations in lissencephaly while acquired intrauterine infections such as CMV and Zika virus also cause cerebral malformations. A wide range of cerebral malformations especially cortical migration defects are seen in children with CP and include: lissencephaly, polymicrogyria, schizencephaly, cortical dysplasia, agenesis of the corpus callosum, holoprosencephaly, and posterior fossa malformations such as Dandy-Walker malformation and Joubert syndrome [19, 38].

Neuroimaging reliably detects cerebral malformations which mainly occur in early gestation thereby implicating antenatal aetiological factors [4]. The detection of cerebral malformation is useful in establishing that the aetiology of CP is unrelated to perinatal events and this may protect the attending Obstetrician from "maternity negligence" claims that are rife in HICs [4, 17].

3.4 Genetic mutations and CP

Genetic aetiology for CP is predictable since CP occurs more frequently in some families/consanguineous families (familial clustering), monozygotic twins and congenital malformations and should be suspected even in those without traditional risk factors [39]. Rare genetic mutations (inherited or de novo) or CP-associated genes are implicated in CP [40, 41]. Indeed, current studies employing new genetic testing techniques called Next Generation Sequencing (NGS) such as whole exome sequencing (WES), whole genome sequencing (WGS) and copy number variant analysis continue to identify pathogenetic variants (copy number variants and single nucleotide variants) and likely pathogenic variants in some cases of CP [40]. For instance, some implicated gene mutations (pathogenic variants) involve KANK1, AP4MI, GAD1, ZC4H2 genes [17, 41]. CP genomics is currently evolving and the discovery of more CP-associated genes or genetic mutations underlying CP is expected to add to the presently known panel of pathogenic variants [41].

The neuropathology of genetic mutations in CP stems directly from disrupting early brain development (specifically motor development) (cerebral malformation) and indirectly through genetic susceptibility to different pathways that cause different neuropathologies [41]. These different pathways include infection/inflammatory cytokine responses, foetal growth restriction/IUGR, prematurity or perinatal stroke since genetic susceptibility has been reported to underlie these other risk factors [41].

3.5 Foetal growth restriction (FGR) and CP

Birth weights below the tenth percentile (10th centile) for gestational age (GA) (small-for-gestational age; SGA) remains a major aetiological/risk factor for CP in both term and preterm babies as shown by multiple studies [42–44]. The risk of CP has been reported to increase with increasing severity of foetal growth restriction (FGR) with babies below the 3rd centile having the greatest risk [44]. However, it has been shown that the large for gestational age (LGA) baby also has increased risk of CP [44]. Recall that macrosomic babies have higher risks related to maternal diabetes and obstructed labour [27] FGR acts indirectly to damage the developing brain through chronic hypoxia-ischaemia resulting from impaired placental function (utero-placental insufficiency) and increased occurrence of perinatal asphyxia and hypoglycaemia [27, 32, 33] (see **Figures 3** and **4**). Thus the neuropathology includes grey matter and WMI (PVL).

3.6 Multiple pregnancy/births and CP

Twinning and higher-order births (triplets, quadruplets, quintuplets, sextuplets, septuplets) from natural or spontaneous conception and Assisted Reproductive Technology (ART) are well-known risks factors for both cerebral dysgenesis and CP [45, 46]. Indeed, the risk of CP increases with increasing number of infants [46]. Peterson et al. [46] in a study of multiple births in Western Australia reported prevalence of CP of 1.6, 7.3 and 28 per 1000 live births in singletons, twins and triplets respectively. The increased risk of CP in multiple births is a consequence of the increased odds of congenital malformations, placental vascular anomalies, FGR, low birth weight (LBW), preterm birth, co-twin death and birth complications/asphyxia (see **Figure 3**) [19, 27, 46]. More so, the increased risk of CP among co-twins has been attributed partly to monochorionic placentation and in-utero death of the co-twin. The "dissolving" or "disappearing twin" is said to release thromboplastin and emboli that can damage the brain of the surviving twin (disappearing twin syndrome) [19, 27, 46]. But a more common setting for brain injury in monochorionic twins by ischaemia and infarctions is the twin-twin transfusion syndrome (TTTS) that results from abnormal placental vascular anastomoses (A-V connections) in which placental tissue supplied by an artery from a donor twin is drained by a vein from the recipient twin [19, 27, 46].

The increasing rate of multiple births reported in HICs suggests an increasing contribution of multiple births to CP pathogenesis [46]. However, a recent large population-cohort study based on Surveillance for Cerebral Palsy in Europe (SCPE) registers found a decreasing risk of CP among the multiples despite the increased prevalence since the 1990s [47]. This study [47] further reported that multiples displayed similar severity of motor impairment as singletons and concluded that advances in obstetric care accounted for these changes in CP risk among preterm low birth weight multiples.

Patently, the neuropathologies of multiple births are the indirect effects on the brain of prematurity, FGR, congenital malformations and hypoxic-ischaemic injury and cerebral infarctions (intrauterine stroke) to which multiples are predisposed (see **Figure 3**).

3.7 Birth/perinatal asphyxia, hypoxic-ischaemic encephalopathy (HIE) or neonatal encephalopathy and CP

Earlier in the discussion, very important facts concerning birth/perinatal asphyxia, HIE and birth complications have been mentioned owing to their significance and the abundance of studies and discussions on them in the literature. Here, a highlight of the definitions/subtle differences between these terms and the neuropathology of neonatal encephalopathy (NE) are emphasized.

Hypoxaemia means a diminished amount of oxygen in the blood supply and at the cellular level while ischaemia is insufficient perfusion; in this context, insufficient cerebral blood flow (CBF) [48]. Ischaemia is usually but not necessarily preceded or accompanied by hypoxia at the cellular level and so the combined term hypoxic-ischaemic injury is applied to describe the combined effect of ischaemia and hypoxia in causing cerebral damage (HIE) [48]. Asphyxia ("suffocation") implies an impairment of respiratory gas exchange accompanied by increased PCO_2, decreased PO_2 (hypoxia) and acidosis. In the early stages of asphyxia, the increased PCO_2 increases CBF through vasodilatory effects on cerebral arteries while later impaired CBF occurs. The ultimate result of ischaemia, hypoxia and or asphyxia is cell death/neuronal necrosis (cerebral damage) through deprivation of O_2 and glucose and energy depletion [48]. When asphyxial events occur in the first or second stage of labour, it is strictly referred to as "birth asphyxia" but "perinatal" or "peripartum asphyxia" is a preferred term since it encompasses foetal or maternal prepartum conditions that predispose to intrapartum hypoxic injury, intrapartum hypoxic injury (birth asphyxia) and the postpartum period of resuscitation for compromised babies with low APGAR scores [49]. Indeed, a failure to initiate and or sustain breathing at birth (birth asphyxia) may originate in the peripartum period (shortly before, during and immediately after birth) with antecedents further upstream in the antenatal period. The latter concept gave birth to the term "Neonatal Encephalopathy" (NE) which is broader than the other terms and has better correlation with CP and long-term neurodevelopmental outcome than birth or perinatal asphyxia that is usually not confirmed in most studies [49].

According to the 2014 report of the American College of Obstetricians and Gynaecologists' (ACOG) Task Force on Neonatal Encephalopathy, Neonatal encephalopathy is a clinically defined syndrome of disturbed neurologic function in the earliest days of life in an infant born at or beyond 35 weeks of gestation, manifested by a subnormal level of consciousness or seizures, and often accompanied by difficulty with initiating and maintaining respiration and depression of tone and reflexes [50]. Thus hypoxic-ischaemic injury (HIE) is only one cause of NE though a significant one. Indeed, a wide range of metabolic, dysgenetic and infectious disorders in the antepartum and postpartum periods also result in NE or are risk factors for NE [49, 50]. Most risk factors for NE are antepartum risk factors [49, 50].

In the literature, one clearly identified challenge is determining with certainty that an intrapartum hypoxic ischaemic injury is responsible for NE or HIE except in few cases when there is a clinically recognized sentinel event like abruptio placentae, umbilical cord prolapse, ruptured uterus, maternal cardiac arrest or amniotic fluid embolus [49, 50]. In view of this, in 2014 the ACOG published criteria for confirming NE due to an acute peripartum or intrapartum event. The neonatal signs reported to be consistent with acute peripartum or intrapartum event are: [50].

a. APGAR scores of <5 at 5 and 10 minutes

b. Foetal umbilical artery academia (pH < 7.0 &/or base deficit ≥12 mmol/L

c. Neuroimaging (MRI or magnetic resonance spectroscopy [MRS]) evidence of acute brain injury consistent with hypoxic-ischaemic injury,

d. Presence of multisystem organ failure (cardiac dysfunction, metabolic & haematologic abnormalities, hepatic, renal & gastrointestinal injuries) consistent with HIE.

However, the presence of other significant risk factors such as maternal infection, IUGR/FGR, foetomaternal haemorrhage, chronic placental lesions and neonatal sepsis makes it unlikely that an acute intrapartum event is the sole underlying pathogenesis of NE [50].

In the earlier report in 2003, the criteria required to define an acute intrapartum hypoxic event as sufficient to cause CP were: [51].

a. Evidence of a metabolic acidosis in foetal umbilical cord arterial blood obtained at delivery (pH < 7.0 & base deficit ≥ 12 mmol/L)

b. Early onset of severe or moderate NE in infants of 34 or more weeks of gestation

c. CP of the spastic quadriplegic (spastic bilateral) or dyskinetic type

d. Exclusion of other identifiable aetiologies such as trauma, coagulation disorders, infectious conditions or genetic disorders.

Obviously, the pivotal role of neuroimaging in delineating brain lesions from diverse aetiologies in CP is recognized by its inclusion in the more recent criteria by ACOG. The neuropathology of NE, though variable depending on gestational age, nature of insult and type of intervention, includes the following predominant patterns of injury in term infants identified by MRI: [49, 52].

- Selective neuronal necrosis: This is the most common injury pattern and involves widespread neuronal necrosis/loss in a characteristic distribution depending on severity and temporal characteristics of the insult. With very severe and very prolonged insults, there is global or diffuse neuronal injury; that is, all levels of the neuraxis (cerebral cortex, basal ganglia, thalamus, brain stem and anterior horn cells of the spinal cord) are affected and the usual long-term sequelae are severe spastic bilateral CP (spastic quadriplegia) with many accompanying impairments due to widespread neuronal injury. The anterior horn cell injury ("hypoxic-ischaemic myelopathy") may explain the characteristic persistence of hypotonia into the first months of life and when severe the unusual persistence into childhood of hypotonia and weakness—the so-called "atonic CP" with atonic quadriparesis. With moderately severe and prolonged insults, cerebral cortex-deep nuclear (cerebral neocortex, hippocampus, basal ganglia [putamen] and thalamus) injury occurs while severe but abrupt insults cause deep nuclear-brainstem (basal ganglia [putamen]-thalamus and brainstem nuclei) injury. The cerebral cortical injury is most prominent in the perirolandic cortex and depths of sulci while the deep nuclear grey matter injury is most prominent in the thalamus and putamen with the intervening posterior limb of the internal capsule (PLIC) affected in moderate or severe thalamo-putaminal injury. In basal nuclei-thalamic injury, neuronal loss, gliosis and hypermyelination in the putamen and thalamus may evolve into status marmoratus (marbled appearance). The basal ganglia-thalamic lesions (BGTL) explain the occurrence of dyskinetic (dystonic/choreoathetoid) CP in NE/HIE (severe perinatal asphyxia) with manifestations of abnormal involuntary movements, tone variability and relatively spared intellectual functions due to the cortical sparing.

- Parasagittal cerebral injury ("watershed infarcts"): This refers to bilateral cerebral cortical and subcortical white matter ischaemic lesions in the parasagittal and superomedial aspects of the cerebral convexities (in the arterial end/border zones or "watershed areas").

- PVL (CWMI): apparently similar to "non-cystic" PVL of very premature infants.

In encephalopathy of prematurity, the main neuropathological feature remains PVL with additional intraventricular haemorrhage with or without periventricular haemorrhagic infarction [31]. The ultimate consequence of PVL is delayed/impaired myelination of cerebral white matter and secondary dysmaturation of grey matter structures such as cortex, thalamus and cerebellum [31].

It is important to note that although MRI best defines the nature and extent of cerebral injury in NE, it is severely limited in determining the aetiology of hypoxic-ischaemic injury and the exact timing of the insult [49, 52]. This may partly explain the apparent contradiction of findings of MRI studies with earlier reports of epidemiological studies [49]. Epidemiologic studies suggest that 70% of CP causation are related to chronic antenatal factors while MRI studies suggest that 75% of cerebral injury in CP occur in the perinatal/intrapartum period owing the preponderance of acute injury patterns (acute peripartum lesions) [49]. In the study by Cowan et al. [53], of 245 infants who had an MRI scan after neurological signs and evidence of intrapartum/perinatal asphyxia (("neonatal encephalopathy"), 80% had MRI evidence of acute peripartum lesions consistent with hypoxic-ischaemic injury, only 4% had MRI evidence of antenatal injury, 16% had normal MRI scans and 4% had other disorders like neuromuscular or metabolic disease [53].

3.8 Perinatal stroke and CP

In children, the perinatal period is associated with the highest risk of stroke and its long-term correlate of spastic unilateral CP (spastic hemiplegia) [54]. Both perinatal arterial ischaemic stroke (foetal/intrauterine and neonatal arterial ischaemic stroke) (PAIS) and cerebral venous sinus thrombosis (CSVT) increase the likelihood of later development of CP [54]. Perinatal ischaemic stroke (PIS) is defined as "a group of heterogeneous conditions in which there is a focal disruption of CBF secondary to arterial or cerebral venous thrombosis or embolization, between 20 weeks of foetal life through twenty-eighth postnatal day confirmed by neuroimaging or neuropathological studies" [55]. Thus, PIS can be of arterial or venous origin (arterial more common), focal or multifocal and occur during intrauterine/prenatal (foetal), intrapartum or postnatal (neonatal) period. In the causation of PAIS, multiple risk factors usually interact [19, 54]. This implies that the pathogenesis of PAIS is multifactorial. The risk factors involved could be maternal, placental or neonatal factors. Some maternal factors include smoking, preeclampsia, thrombophilia, maternal infections and intrapartum complications while neonatal factors are male sex, APGAR score of <7 (5 minutes), prolonged resuscitation, congenital heart disease, thrombophilia, early-onset sepsis/meningitis and vascular abnormality [19, 54]. The placental factors include chorioamnionitis, chronic villitis with obliterative foetal vasculopathy, thrombotic vasculopathy and small placenta (see **Figure 4**) [19, 54].

The neuropathological lesions of PAIS are localized areas of infarction (necrosis of all cellular elements) within the distribution of single (or multiple) major cerebral vessel(s) (specific vascular distribution) and commonly with cavity formation depending on the time of occurrence. Focal and multifocal necroses of brain in the prenatal and early postnatal periods are associated with dissolution of tissue and cavity formation variously termed porencephaly, hydranencephaly and multicystic encephalomalacia which have all been reported by MRI studies on CP [4, 54].

3.9 Unconjugated hyperbilirubinaemia and CP

Severe unconjugated hyperbilirubinaemia remains a significant perinatal/postnatal aetiological factor for CP in LMICs of sub-Saharan Africa and south Asia due to suboptimal management of neonatal jaundice [56, 57]. However, in HICs, kernicterus spectrum disorder (KSD) also occurs especially in preterm/low birth weight babies where brain damage may be present at levels of total serum bilirubin (TSB) below the "safe level" or without signs of acute bilirubin encephalopathy (ABE) (the so-called "low bilirubin kernicterus") [56]. Some causes of unconjugated hyperbilirubinaemia that manifest as ABE and KSD include Rhesus and ABO incompatibilities, G6PD deficiency, prematurity/low birth weight and Crigler-Najjar syndrome type 1 while the risk factors for KSD are: asphyxia, prematurity, low birth weight, acidosis, sepsis, hypoalbuminaemia, hyperthermia and respiratory distress [56–58]. The latter are factors that facilitate bilirubin neurotoxicity (BNTx) by making it easier for the hydrophobic, lipid soluble free or unconjugated bilirubin to cross the blood brain barrier (BBB) to damage specific regions of the brain (selective bilirubin neurotoxicity) [56, 57].

The neuropathology of ABE and KSD comprises bilirubin (yellow) staining of brainstem nuclei ("kernicterus") and neuronal necrosis, loss and gliosis in the basal ganglia/nuclei (Globus pallidus & subthalamic nucleus) and hippocampus [56–58]. Thus, the major areas of neuronal damage (selective bilirubin neurotoxicity) are basal nuclei/ganglia (globus pallidus), subthalamic nucleus of thalamus, oculomotor and cochlear (auditory) brainstem nuclei and the cerebellar dentate and Purkinje cells of the cerebellum in preterm infants [8, 56–58]. On MRI, the main findings in ABE are bilateral and symmetrical abnormalities (hyperintensities) of Globus pallidus and subthalamic nucleus (rarely hippocampus) on T_1 and T_2-weighted images [4]. These neuropathological substrates underlie the clinical manifestations of dyskinetic CP (basal ganglia injury) and the accompanying impairments of sensorineural deafness (cochlear/auditory nuclear damage), gaze palsies (brainstem CN III, IV, VI nuclear damage) in kernicterus [56–58].

3.10 Meningitis/meningoencephalitis, cerebral malaria and CP

Preventable postnatal risk factors for CP are more prevalent in LMICs than HICs and include bacterial meningitis, meningoencephalitis and cerebral malaria [3, 59–61]. In a population-based study in Uganda, cerebral injury resulting in CP was attributed to cerebral malaria/cerebral infections in 25% of cases [60]. Over 90% of cases of cerebral malaria occur in sub-Saharan Africa and in children under 5 years of age [59–61].

In brief, the neuropathology of meningitis/meningoencephalitis comprises diffuse neuronal injury (necroses) and cerebral white matter injury (PVL similar to that of prematurity) through a complex cascade of inflammatory cytokine-mediated damage that leads to cerebral oedema, increased intracranial pressure, decreased CBF, vasculitis and thromboses, ischaemia and infarction [62]. On the contrary, the precise neuropathogenesis of cerebral malaria has not been fully elucidated but a number of theories have been put forward including the "mechanical (sequestration) hypothesis" and the "cytokine storm hypothesis" [63]. In a word, regardless of either vascular obstruction from sequestration of parasitized red blood cells in brain capillaries and venules or cytokine-mediated inflammatory injury, ultimately, cerebral malaria causes grey and white matter damage. Severe spastic bilateral CP specifically spastic quadriplegia is the expected long-term correlate of these postnatal CNS infections since they are diffuse processes with extensive brain damage [64]. Indeed, Iloeje and Ogoke [64] in their study on severity of CP in children found a strong correlation between postnatal CNS infections and severe/non-ambulatory CP. Thus the greater contribution of postnatal CNS infections to CP causation in LMICs may in part be the reason for the relatively poorer gross motor function in children with CP from LMICs compared to their counterparts from HICs [64].

4. Clinico-neuropathological correlations in CP: the "hows and "whys"

The clinical features, clinical subtypes of CP and the accompanying physical, mental and physiological impairments are described here in relation to the aforementioned neuropathological substrates of CP.

4.1 Overview of brain areas and pathways involved in control of posture and movement

The normal control of movement (voluntary and involuntary, gross and fine), maintenance of a stable posture and balance, muscle tone and coordination of motor activity involve intricate interactions between the cerebral motor cortex, basal nuclei/subcortical grey mater (putamen, globus pallidus, subthalamic nucleus, substantial nigra, thalamus), brainstem nuclei (vestibular nucleus, superior colliculus, red nucleus) and cerebellum with the cells of the ventral or anterior horn of the spinal cord (alpha and gamma motor neurons) [65]. On emerging from the anterior horn cells, the motor neurons in peripheral nerves (lower motor neurons [LMN]) innervate the muscles of the body to effect movement/muscle contraction [65]. Each alpha motor neuron and all muscle fibres that it innervates constitute a motor unit—the functional unit of the motor system [65]. Functionally, the descending motor pathways from the brain to spinal cord (upper motor neurons [UMN]) are subdivided into pyramidal and extrapyramidal pathways [65]. The pyramidal pathway arise from the cerebral cortex and send motor signals to the spinal cord (corticospinal tract) and to brainstem nuclei (corticobulbar tract) for voluntary control of muscles of the body and face respectively [65]. The extrapyramidal tracts (vestibulospinal, reticulospinal, rubrospinal, tectospinal tracts) take their origin from different brainstem nuclei and project to the spinal cord for control of involuntary/automatic muscle activity like control of muscle tone through the stretch reflex, posture and movement [65]. The stretch reflex arc for maintenance of muscle tone is controlled by the inhibitory influence of corticospinal and dorsal reticulospinal tracts and facilitatory influence by medial reticulospinal and vestibulospinal tracts [65, 66]. The basal nuclei function to facilitate or fine tune voluntary movement while inhibiting undesired movements and they receive projections from the motor cortex and project back to the motor cortex through the thalamus [65]. Thus, the occurrence of unwanted involuntary movements in basal ganglia injury. The cerebellum is also deeply involved in maintenance of balance, posture and coordination of movement and damage to it produces ataxia [65, 66]. The pyramidal/corticospinal tract is increasingly vulnerable to damage at different points along their long course to the spinal cord and commonly include their site of origin at the cerebral cortex, corona radiata and the white matter (internal capsule) between the thalamus and basal nuclei [65]. This may contribute to the high prevalence of spastic CP and its combination with other forms of CP in the so-called "mixed CP" subtypes such as spastic dystonic CP and combinations of spasticity and choreoathetosis.

4.2 Neuromotor impairments and musculoskeletal deficits in CP

In spastic CP, the brain lesions in the various predominant locations disrupt the descending pyramidal pathways resulting in an UMN syndrome whose primary manifestations are categorized into positive and negative features that act in concert to cause secondary progressive musculoskeletal pathology/impairments [66–68]. The positive features of UMN syndrome are spasticity, hyperreflexia, clonus, co-contraction while the negative features include weakness, loss of selective motor control (SMC), poor balance, fatigability and sensory deficits [66–68]. The positive features result from brain lesions disrupting the facilitatory corticobulbar fibres (from the premotor cortex), thus leading to inhibition of the dorsal reticulospinal tract (from the brainstem ventromedial reticular formation) which exerts inhibitory control over the stretch reflex [66–68]. Spasticity refers to a velocity-dependent increase in muscle tone with exaggerated tendon jerks due to hyperexcitable or increased tonic spinal stretch reflex [65–68]. This implies that the loss of inhibition of the spinal stretch reflex by descending pathways result in overactivity of the spinal stretch reflex and underlies the findings of spasticity, hyperreflexia and clonus in pyramidal CP [66–68]. The voluntary output from the motor cortex activates motor neurons targeting the agonist muscles while simultaneously inhibiting the antagonist muscles through the Ia interneurons (reciprocal inhibition) [66]. It is the loss of this reciprocal inhibition of antagonist muscles during voluntary command that underlies co-contraction and it makes generation of force or movement difficult [66].

In spastic CP, there is significant weakness that contributes to abnormal posture and movement. The weakness is consequent on a number of factors such as reduced muscle size/volume, reduced muscle activation, lower frequency motor unit firing rates and increased Type 1 muscle fibres due to an altered neural input to muscle (reduced neuromuscular activation) caused by the damage to the descending corticospinal tracts [68]. This is also accompanied by decreased muscle endurance and loss of selective motor control (SMC) [67, 68]. Loss of selective motor control is the impaired ability to single out the activation of specific muscles in response to demands of a voluntary posture or movement [67, 68]. For example, the co-activation of quadriceps femoris (knee extension) and gastrocnemius (ankle planter flexion) in a child with severe spastic CP [68]. The weakness, impaired SMC and poor balance (negative features) are pivotal in determining when or if a child with CP will walk [67, 68]. It is also important to note that some surgical interventions for spasticity such as muscle lengthening, tendon transfer, selective dorsal rhizotomy and intrathecal baclofen all reduce muscle strength while orthoses and serial casting may worsen weakness through immobilization [67, 68]. The reduced descending excitatory signals on muscle growth results in impaired muscle growth (smaller muscles) and a short muscle-tendon unit which contributes to muscle weakness in spastic CP("short muscle disease") [67, 68]. The failure of muscle growth to progress at same speed with bone growth (muscle-to-bone growth rate discrepancy) which is more prominent in bi-articular muscles like rectus femoris, hamstrings and gastrocnemius underlies the joint contractures and gait abnormalities such as toe-walking and flexed-knee gait in spastic CP [67, 68].

In non-spastic or extrapyramidal CP with damage to the basal nuclei, the clinical manifestations are abnormal, involuntary, uncontrolled, recurrent and occasionally stereotyped movements with fluctuating tone and persistence of primitive reflexes [68]. In dystonia, there are involuntary sustained or intermittent muscle contractions of both agonist and antagonist muscles causing twisting and repetitive movements and or abnormal postures with increased tone [65–68]. Choreoathetosis is characterized by a combination of random-appearing sequence of one or more discrete, excessive and rapid movements or fragment of movement of proximal body parts/trunk (chorea) with slow, continuous, writhing movements of distal body parts that impedes maintenance of a stable posture (athetosis) [65–68]. Both dystonic and choreoathetoid movements impair function [68].

However, the terms spastic (pyramidal) and extrapyramidal CP are strictly incorrect [5, 65]. It is more accurate to refer to these as "predominantly spastic" and "predominantly non-spastic" [65] . Due to the complex interactions of the upper motor neuron system (the pyramidal, extrapyramidal and cerebellar pathways) with anterior horn cells to control posture and movement, lesions causing CP in real life usually involve both pyramidal and extrapyramidal pathways [65]. This explains the clinical combination of motor/movement abnormalities such as spasticity with dystonia, and spasticity with choreoathetosis ("mixed CP"). Thus, the mixed CP subtype should actually be very common but spastic CP remains the commonest type thereby exposing the subjectivity and imprecision in assessment of patients based on the physiologic classification of CP [2, 69].

In the rare ataxic CP with damage to the cerebellum, clinical features are hypotonia, limb incoordination, and poor balance and these result in instability and a compensatory wide base of support with elevated, outstretched arm postures to improve balance during gait (ataxia) [65, 68].

Therefore, the primary neurologic correlates of early brain injury in CP include: [2, 66–68].

- Delayed developmental milestones; invariably and most severely affecting the motor domain

- Abnormalities of movement or motor patterns, muscle tone and reflex patterns including persistence of primitive reflexes

- Abnormalities of gait and posture ranging from toe-walking to crouched gait

- Muscle weakness, poor balance, impaired selective motor control

- Incoordination and ataxia

4.3 Secondary impairments and accompanying disorders in CP

The accompanying physical, mental or physiological impairments identified in the current definition of CP include epilepsy, cognitive impairment (intellectual disability), speech, visual and hearing impairments and secondary musculoskeletal pathology [1]. These secondary or accompanying impairments are significant since they may cause more functional limitation than the primary motor dysfunction (the core feature of CP) [1, 2].

4.3.1 Epilepsy

Epilepsy is a chronic brain disease characterized by two or more unprovoked or reflex seizures more than 24 hours apart or presence of an epilepsy syndrome [70]. Epilepsy remains a common accompanying disorder in CP occurring in 30–60% of children diagnosed with CP [71, 72]. Both CP and epilepsy in most cases arise from the same underlying neuropathological substrate [71]. Cerebral dysgenesis (disorders of cortical malformation like lissencephaly, cortical dysplasia, heterotopias, corpus callosal agenesis), cortical infarctions (perinatal stroke and meningoencephalitis) and diffuse cortical neuronal necrosis (severe neonatal encephalopathy/HIE) are neuropathological substrates for both CP and epilepsy [71]. Thus the aetiology of epilepsy in CP could be structural (cerebral dysgenesis, infarctions, postnatal head trauma), postinfectious (CMV, Toxoplasmosis, post meningoencephalitis) or genetic [70]. The latter occurs in cases of CP who on newer genetic testing techniques (WES, WGS) also show genetic or copy number variants pathogenic for epilepsy with or without a family history of epilepsy [70]. Epilepsies in CP are more common in spastic quadriplegia and hemiplegia owing to the cerebral cortical involvement in spastic quadriplegia and hemiplegia and are relatively uncommon in spastic diplegia due to the relative sparing of the cortex in PVL of prematurity [71–73].

It has been reported that epilepsy is more prevalent in severe CP/GMFCS levels IV-V and in the presence of co-morbid intellectual disability (ID) [72]. These findings most likely relate to the degree/topography of cortical injury since diffuse cortical neuronal necrosis (SNN) from severe neonatal encephalopathy/HIE or cortical malformations result in spastic quadriplegia that is usually associated with severe gross motor dysfunction (non-ambulatory status) [2, 49].

4.3.2 Cognitive deficits/intellectual disability (ID), behavioural, attentional and socialization defects

The ID that occurs in severe CP is a consequence of mainly the cerebral cortical injury with injury to the basal nuclei, thalamus and cerebellum playing an additional role [49]. Intellectual retardation almost invariably accompanies the diffuse variety of selective neuronal necrosis (SNN) in severe NE/HIE in term infants [49]. In preterm infants, intellectual function is more severely affected (significantly lower intelligence quotients [IQ]) in those with spastic quadriplegia than spastic diplegia [32]. In the PVL of encephalopathy of prematurity, more severe lesions with lateral extension into the centrum semiovale and corona radiata would be expected to affect upper extremities in addition (spastic quadriplegia) and intellectual functions as well [32]. The primary white matter injury in encephalopathy of prematurity leads to secondary dysmaturation of grey matter structures with widespread reduction in cerebral volumes (cerebral cortex, deep nuclear grey matter, hippocampus, total cerebral tissue and cerebellum) [32]. White matter injury also underlies the deficits in executive function, behavioural disturbances and socialization deficits and partly explains why language delay, Attention Deficit Hyperactivity Disorder (ADHD) and Autism Spectrum Disorder (ASD) may accompany CP especially in children born prematurely [32]. Hyperactivity and inattention may in part be due to involvement of neurons of the reticular activating system (RAS), the basal nuclei or the cerebellum [32].

4.3.3 Visual abnormalities/squints and cortical visual impairments

Ptosis, oculomotor and gaze abnormalities result primarily from disturbance or injury to brainstem cranial nerve (CN) nuclei (CN III, IV, VI, VII). in the deep nuclear-brainstem variety of SNN associated with severe and abrupt hypoxic-ischaemic insults in term infants. Severe diffuse cortical necrosis (SNN) involving the visual or occipital cortex underlies impairment of cortical visual functions in children with CP since many of them have cerebral cortical atrophy [49]. Nevertheless, in prematurity, visual impairment could be a consequence of retinopathy of prematurity or injury to white matter visual pathways (PVL) (cerebral visual impairment [CVI]) [32]. PVL is strongly associated with visual impairment since the principal area of injury includes the optic radiations (geniculocalcarine tracts) and visual association areas [32]. This implies that more severe PVL with more extensive lesions involving the peritrigonal white matter, optic radiations and occipital cortex correlates with poorer future vision [32].

4.3.4 Hearing and speech deficits, feeding difficulties and undernutrition

Brainstem CN nuclear involvement in severe NE/HIE underlies the accompanying feeding difficulties due to poor coordination and impairments of sucking (CN V), swallowing (CN IX & X) and tongue movements (CN XII) [49]. It is also possible that in addition to the nuclear injury (bulbar palsy), corticobulbar disturbance (pseudobulbar palsy) contributes to these deficits [49]. The ultimate consequences of the feeding difficulties in young children with CP are undernutrition and stunting unless alternative means of feeding like gastrostomy are employed. However, some well-fed non-ambulatory children with CP may become overweight due to the imbalance between energy intake and utilization.

Oral-motor-dysfunction (from bulbar and or pseudobulbar palsy) causes speech deficits due to weakness and poor coordination of the muscles innervated by CN V, VII, IX, X and XII that are involved in speech and phonation. Injury to the dorsal cochlear nuclei and or cochlea, superior olivary nucleus and inferior colliculus result in hearing deficits in CP [49]. Free or unconjugated bilirubin damages the brainstem auditory nuclei and auditory nerve (bilirubin neurotoxicity) in auditory neuropathy spectrum disorders with or without sensorineural hearing loss (ANSD). This explains the common co-morbid sensorineural deafness in dyskinetic CP secondary to chronic bilirubin encephalopathy (Kernicterus spectrum disorders) [56, 57].

4.3.5 Musculoskeletal problems, gait abnormalities and pain

The musculoskeletal pathology such as muscle shortening/contracture, bony torsion, joint instability, premature degenerative arthritis in weight-bearing joints are secondary to the integrated effects of the positive and negative features of the UMN syndrome in CP [67, 68]. These musculoskeletal problems and the resultant gait abnormalities and pain are progressive as they worsen over time without early intervention [67, 68]. As children with CP grow, the growth of bone outpaces that of the skeletal muscle resulting in contractures such as gastrocnemius contracture and planter flexed or equinus gait [67, 68]. Thus juveniles develop scoliosis, hip dislocation/subluxation, and fixed contractures as growth spurts occur [67, 68]. Immobility contributes to the pathogenesis of the musculoskeletal abnormalities and explains in part the increased frequency of orthopaedic complications in children with severe gross motor dysfunction or non-ambulatory CP (spastic quadriplegia/Gross Motor Function Classification [GMFCS] levels IV/V) [67, 68].

5. Conclusions

The aetiology of CP is attributed to the interaction of multiple risk factors which through complex causal pathways within a limited duration disrupt brain development or augment the risk of damage to the motor system in the foetal/infant brain. It has remained a challenge to identify with certainty the timing of these non-progressive disturbances. Nevertheless, the increasing role of genetic susceptibility in CP causation is evolving.

A link between neuropathology and the clinical-neurological features of CP (neuromuscular deficits, accompanying impairments, severity/functional level, clinical types) exists. However, limitations currently remain in devising a comprehensive neuropathologic classification of CP due to inconsistent structure-function correlations and difficulties in estimating timing of insults. Overall, a gap currently exists in our understanding of the aetiology and pathogenesis of CP despite the pivotal roles of advanced neuroimaging and evolving genomics.

Acknowledgements

I express my deep appreciation to my supervisor Dr. Abdul Hawas Manshour for his assistance and Dr. Ahmed Shamakhi and the staff of Department of Paediatrics at the King Fahd Central Hospital, Jazan, for their support by providing me a platform to deepen my knowledge and practice of Paediatric Neurology. I am indebted too to my beautiful "Finebaby"—Mrs. Linda Chigozie Ogoke whose sweet love and support sustained me during the period of writing up of this book chapter.

Conflict of interest

None.

Author details

Christian Chukwukere Ogoke
Consultant Paediatric Neurologist, Paediatric Neurology Unit, Department of Paediatrics, King Fahd Central Hospital, Jizan, Saudi Arabia

*Address all correspondence to: chrischikere@yahoo.com

References

[1] Bax M, Goldstein M, Rosenbaum P, Paneth N. Proposed definition and classification of cerebral palsy. Developmental Medicine and Child Neurology. 2005;**47**:571-576. DOI: 10.1017/s001216220500112x

[2] Ogoke CC. Clinical classification of cerebral palsy. In: Al-Zwaini IJ, editor. Cerebral Palsy—Clinical and Therapeutic Aspects. London, United Kingdom: IntechOpen; 2018. DOI: 10.5772/intechopen.79246. ISBN:978-1-78984-831-1

[3] Reddihough DS, Collins KJ. The epidemiology and causes of cerebral palsy. The Australian Journal of Physiotherapy. 2003;**49**:7-12

[4] Korzeniewski SJ, Birbeck G, Delano MC, Potchen MJ, Paneth N. A systematic review of neuroimaging for cerebral palsy. Journal of Child Neurology. 2008;**23**(2):218-227. DOI: 10.1177/0883073807307983

[5] Pakula AT, Braun KVN, Yeargin-Allsopp M. Cerebral palsy: Classification and epidemiology. Physical Medicine and Rehabilitation Clinics of North America. 2009;**20**:425-452

[6] Rosenbaum PL, Paneth N, Leviton A, Goldstein M, Bax M. The definition and classification of cerebral palsy. Developmental Medicine and Child Neurology. 2007;**49**(8):1-44

[7] Yokochi K, Fujimoto S. Magnetic resonance imaging in children with neonatal asphyxia: Correlation with developmental sequalae. Acta Paediatrica. 1996;**85**:88-95

[8] Johnston MV, Hoon AH. Possible mechanisms in infants for selective basal ganglia damage from asphyxia, kernicterus, or mitochondrial encephalopathies. Journal of Child Neurology. 2000;**15**:588-591

[9] Nelson KB, Ellenberg JH. Antecedents of cerebral palsy,1. Univariate analysis of risks. American Journal of Diseases of Children. 1985;**139**:1031-1038

[10] Nelson KB, Ellenberg JH. Antecedents of cerebral palsy. Multivariate analysis of risk. New England Journal of Medicine. 1986;**315**(2):81-86. DOI: 10.1056/NEJM198607103150202

[11] Himmelmann K, Ahlin K, Jacobsson B, Cans C, Thorsen P. Risk factors for cerebral palsy in children born at term. Acta Obstetricia et Gynecologica Scandinavica. 2011;**90**(10):1070-1081. DOI: 10.1111/j.1600-0412.2011.0127.x.Epub 2011 jul 27

[12] Suvanand S, Kapoor SK, Reddaiah VP, Singh U, Sundaram KR. Risk factors for cerebral palsy. Indian Journal of Pediatrics. 1997;**64**(5):677-685

[13] Ahlin K, Himmelmann K, Hagberg G, Kacerovsky M, Cobo T, Wennerholm UB, et al. Non-infectious risk factors for different types of cerebral palsy in term-born babies: A population-based, case-control study. BJOG : An International Journal of Obstetrics and Gynaecology. 2013;**120**(6):724-731

[14] Solemani F, Vamegh R, Biglarian A. Antenatal and intrapartum risk factors for cerebral palsy in term and near-term newborns. Archives of Iranian Medicine. 2013;**16**(4):213-216

[15] Adogu P, Ubajaka CF, Egenti NP, Obinwa AM, Igwe W. Evaluation of risk factors of cerebral palsy in tertiary health facility, Nnewi, Nigeria: A case-control

study. International Journal of Medical Science and Public Health. 2016;**5**(1):1-7

[16] Korzeniewski Steven J, Romero R, Cortez J, Pappas A, Schwartz Alyse G, Kim Chong J, et al. A "multi-hit" model of neonatal white matter injury: Cumulative contributions of chronic placental inflammation, acute fetal inflammation and postnatal inflammatory events. Journal of Perinatal Medicine. 2014;**42**(6):731-743

[17] MacLennan AH, Thompson SC. Cerebral palsy: Causes, pathways, and the role of genetic variants. American Journal of Obstetrics & Gynecology. 2015;**213**(6):779-788. DOI: 10.1016/j.ajog.2015.05.034

[18] Stanley FJ, Blair E, Alberman E. Cerebral palsies: Epidemiology and causal pathways. In: Clinics in Developmental Medicine. Vol. 51. London: Mackeith Press; 2000

[19] Korzeniewsky SJ, Slaughter J, Lenski M, Haak P, Paneth N. The complex aetiology of cerebral palsy. Nature Reviews Neurology. 2018;**14**:528-543. DOI: 10.1038/s41582-018-0045-6

[20] Kavcic A, Vodusek DB. A historical perspective on cerebral palsy as a concept and a diagnosis. European Journal of Neurology. 2005;**12**:582-587

[21] Nelson KB. What proportion of cerebral palsy is related to birth asphyxia? Journal of Paediatrics. 1998;**112**:572-574

[22] Yoon BH, Jun JK, Romero R. Amniotic fluid inflammatory cytokines (interleukin-6, interleukin-beta, and tumor necrosis factor-alpha), neonatal brain white matter lesions, and cerebral palsy. American Journal of Obstetrics & Gynecology. 1997;**177**:19-26

[23] Nelson KB, Dambrosia JM, Grether JK, Philips TM. Neonatal cytokines and coagulation factors in children with cerebral palsy. Annals of Neurology. 1998;**44**:665-675

[24] Grether JK, Nelson KB, Dambrosia JM, Philips TM. Interferons and cerebral palsy. Journal of Pediatrics. 1999;**134**:324-332

[25] Yoon BH, Romero R, Park JS, et al. Fetal exposure to an intramniotic inflammation and the development of cerebral palsy at the age of three years. American Journal of Obstetrics & Gynecology. 2000;**182**:675-681

[26] Donald KA, Semia P, Kakooza-Mwesige A, Bearden D. Pediatric cerebral palsy in Africa: A systematic review. Seminars in Pediatric Neurology. 2014;**21**:30-35. DOI: 10.1016/j.spen2014.01.001

[27] Eunson P. Aetiology and epidemiology of cerebral palsy. Paediatrics and Child Health. 2012;**22**(9):361-366

[28] van Haastert IC, Groenendaal F, Uiterwaal CS, Termote JU, van der Heide-Jalving M, Eijsermans MJ, et al. Decreasing incidence and severity of cerebral palsy in prematurely born children. The Journal of Pediatrics. 2011;**159**:86-91.e1

[29] Xue J, Chen L, Xue L, Zhou Q. Meta-analysis of risk factors for childhood cerebral palsy during pregnancy. Zhongguo Dang Dai Er Ke Za Zhi. 2013;**15**(7):535-540

[30] Oskoui M, Coutinho F, Dykeman J, Jette E, Pringsheim T. An update on the prevalence of cerebral palsy: A systematic review and meta-analysis. Developmental Medicine and Child Neurology. 2013;**55**:509-519

[31] Kinney HC, Volpe JJ. Encephalopathy of prematurity: Neuropathology. In: Volpe's Neurology of the Newborn. 6th ed. Philadelphia, PA: Elsevier. pp. 389-404

[32] Neil JJ, Volpe JJ. Encephalopathy of prematurity: Clinical-neurological features, diagnosis, imaging, prognosis, therapy. In: Volpe's Neurology of the Newborn. 6th ed. Philadelphia, PA: Elsevier. pp. 425-457

[33] Neufeld M, Frigon C, Graham A, et al. Maternal infection and risk of cerebral palsy in term and preterm infants. Journal of Perinatology. 2005;**25**:108-113

[34] Mcintyre S, Taitz D, Keogh J, Goldsmith S, Badawi N, Blair E. A systematic review of risk factors for cerebral palsy in children born at term in developed countries. Developmental Medicine & Child Neurology. 2013;**55**:499-508

[35] Ayubi E, Sarhadi S, Mansori K. Maternal infection during pregnancy and risk of cerebral palsy in children: A systematic review and meta-analysis. Journal of Child Neurology. 2021;**36**(5):385-402

[36] Wu YW, Colford JM Jr. Chorioamnionitis as a risk factor for cerebral palsy: A meta-analysis. JAMA. 2000;**284**(11):1417-1424

[37] Hermansen MC, Hermansen MG. Perinatal infections and cerebral palsy. Clinics in Perinatology. 2006;**33**:315-333

[38] Hoon AH Jr. Neuroimaging in cerebral palsy: Patterns of brain dysgenesis and injury. Journal of Child Neurology. 2005;**12**:936-939

[39] Schaefer GB. Genetic considerations in cerebral palsy. Pediatric Neurology. 2008;**15**:21-26

[40] Moreno-de-Luca A, Millan F, Pesacreta DR, et al. Molecular diagnostic yield of exome sequencing in patients with cerebral palsy. JAMA. 2021;**325**(5):467-475

[41] Lewis SA, Shetty S, Wilson BA, Huang AJ, et al. Insights from genetic studies of cerebral palsy. Frontiers in Neurology. 2021;**11**:625428

[42] Zhao M, Dai H, Deng Y, Zhao L. SGA as a risk factor for cerebral palsy in moderate to late preterm infants: A system review and meta-analysis. Scientific Reports. 2016;**6**:38853

[43] Jarvis S, Glinianala SV, Torrioli M, Platt M, Miceli M, Jouk P, et al. Cerebral palsy and intrauterine growth in single births. European collaborative study. Lancet. 2003;**362**:1106-1111

[44] O'Callaghan ME, MacLennan AH, Gibson CS, et al. Epidemiologic associations with cerebral palsy. Obstetrics and Gynecology. 2011;**118**:576-582

[45] Bonellie S, Currie D, Chalmers J. Comparison of risk factors for cerebral palsy in twins and singletons. Developmental Medicine and Child Neurology. 2005;**47**(09):345-351

[46] Petterson B, Nelson KB, Watson L, Stanley F. Twins, triplets, and cerebral palsy in births in Western Australia in the 1980s. BMJ. 1993;**307**(6914):1239-1243

[47] Perra O, Rankin J, Platt MJ, et al. Decreasing cerebral palsy prevalence in multiple births in the modern era: a population cohort study of European data. Archives of Disease in Childhood. Fetal and Neonatal Edition. 2021;**106**:F125-F130

[48] Inder TE, Volpe JJ. Hypoxic Ischaemic and related disorders: Pathophysiology:

General principles. In: Volpe's Neurology of the Newborn. 6th ed. Philadelphia, PA: Elsevier. pp. 325-388

[49] Inder TE, Volpe JJ. Hypoxic-Ischaemic injury in the term infant: Clinical–neurological features, diagnosis, imaging, prognosis, therapy. In: Volpe's Neurology of the Newborn. 6th ed. Philadelphia, PA: Elsevier. pp. 510-563

[50] American College of Obstetricians and Gynecologists. Execurive summary: Neonatal encephalopathy and neurologic outcome. Obstetrics and Gynecology. 2014;**123**:896-901

[51] Neonatal Encephalopathy and cerebral palsy. Defining the pathogenesis and pathophysiology: A report. Obstetrics and Gynecology. 2003;**102**(3):628-636

[52] Kinney HC, Volpe JJ. Hypoxic-Ischaemic injury in the term infant: Neuropathology. In: Volpe's Neurology of the Newborn. 6th ed. Philadelphia, PA: Elsevier. pp. 484-499

[53] Cowan F, Rutherford M, Groenendaal F, et al. Origin and timing of brain lesions in term infants with neonatal encephalopathy. Lancet. 2003;**361**:736-742

[54] Inder TE, Volpe JJ. Stroke in the newborn. In: Volpe's Neurology of the Newborn. 6th ed. Philadelphia, PA: Elsevier. pp. 510-563

[55] Raju TN, Nelson KB, Ferriero D, et al. Ischaemic perinatal stroke: Summary of a workshop sponsored by the National Institute of Child Health and Human Development and the National Institute of neurological disorders and stroke. Pediatrics. 2007;**120**(3):609-616

[56] Jayanti S, Ghersi-Egea J, Strazielle N, Tiribelli C, Gazzin S. Severe neonatal hyperbilirubinaemia and the brain: The old but still evolving story. Pediatric Medicine. 2021;**4**:37

[57] Riordan SM, Shapiro SM. Review of bilirubin toxicity I: Molecular biology and neuropathology of disease. Pediatric Research. 2020;**87**:327-331

[58] Gamber AC, Toth EM, Vreman HJ, Slusher TM. Neonatal hyperbilirubinaemia in low –medium income African countries. International Journal of Pediatric Research. 2021;**7**:073

[59] Gladstone M. A review of the incidence and prevalence, types and aetiology of childhood cerebral palsy in resource-poor settings. Annals of Tropical Paediatrics. 2010;**30**:181-196

[60] Kakooza-Mwesige A, Andrews C, Peterson S, Mangen FW, Eliasson AC, Forssberg H. Prevalence of cerebral palsy in Uganda: A population-based study. The Lancet Global Health. 2017;**5**:e1275-e1282

[61] Duke R, Torty C, Nwachukwu K, et al. Clinical features and aetiology of cerebral palsy in children from Cross River state, Nigeria. Archives of Disease in Childhood. 2020;**105**:625-630

[62] de Vries LS, Volpe JJ. Bacterial and fungal intracranial infections. In: Volpe's Neurology of the Newborn. 6th ed. Philadelphia, PA: Elsevier. pp. 1050-1089

[63] Schiess N, Villabona-Rueda A, Cottier KE, Huether K, Chipeta J, Stins MF. Pathophysiology and neurologic sequelae of cerebral malaria. Malaria Journal. 2020;**19**:266

[64] Iloeje SO, Ogoke CC. Factors associated with severity of motor impairment in children with cerebral palsy seen in Enugu, Nigeria. South African Journal of Child Health. 2017;**11**(3):112-116

[65] Ganong WF. Control of posture and movement. In: Review of Medical Physiology. 22nd ed. Singapore: McGraw-Hill; 2005. pp. 202-222

[66] Trompetto C, Marinelli L, Mori L, Pelosin E, Curra A, Molfetta L, et al. Pathophysiology of spasticity: Implications for neurorehabilitation. BioMed Research International. 2014;**354906**:1-9

[67] Graham HK, Selber P. Musculoskeletal aspects of cerebral palsy. Journal of Bone and Joint Surgery. [British Volume]. 2003;**85-B**:157-166

[68] Zhou J, Butler EE, Rose J. Neurologic correlates of gait abnormalities in cerebral palsy: Implications for treatment. Frontiers in Human Neuroscience. 2017;**11**:103

[69] Sellier E, Platt MJ, Anderson GL, Krågeloh-Mann I, De La Cruz J, Cans C. Decreasing prevalence in cerebral palsy: A multi-site European population-based study, 1980 to 2003. Developmental Medicine and Child Neurology. 2016;**58**:85-92

[70] Falco-Walter JJ, Scheffer IE, Fisher RS. The new definition and classification of seizures and epilepsy. Epilepsy Research. 2018;**139**:73-79

[71] Jekovec-Vrhovsek M. Epilepsy in children with cerebral palsy. Eastern Journal of Medicine. 2012;**17**:166-170

[72] Bruck I, Antoniuk SA, Spessato A, de Bem RS, Hausberger R, Pacheco CG. Epilepsy in children with cerebral palsy. Arquivos de Neuro-Psiquiatria. 2001;**59**(1):35-39

[73] Lin J-P. The cerebral palsies: A physiologic approach. Journal of Neurology, Neurosurgery, and Psychiatry. 2003;**74**(Suppl I):i23-i29

Section 2

Treatment of Cerebral Palsy

Chapter 2

Management of Spasticity and Cerebral Palsy Update

Yasser Awaad

Abstract

Cerebral palsy is a very common medical problem, which has many challenges facing patients, family, caregivers, and medical team. The fast-based technology helped us to find new ways to manage and treat cerebral palsy. Treatment and management is a multi-disciplinary approach to reaching the optimal results. The managing team includes a general pediatrician, pediatric neurologist, pediatric rehabilitation, pediatric neurosurgeon, pediatric orthopedic surgeon, and other ancillary medical services. In our management plan, we have to consider the patient, family, and caregivers as parts of our plan. Raising awareness in the communities especially young mothers and general pediatricians to recognize the problem early and seek medical help and also early referrals to specialized centers will help to have early intervention and obtain better results.

Keywords: management, spasticity, cerebral palsy, treatment, update

1. Introduction

The focus of this chapter is the management of spasticity in CP children by demonstrating the different treatment options available to the child and his/her family. Spasticity was defined by Lance as a "velocity-dependent increase in tonic stretch reflexes (muscle tone) with exaggerated tendon jerks, resulting from hyperexcitability of the stretch reflex [1].

Treatment for spasticity was documented as early as the late nineteenth century when surgeons Abbe and Bennet discussed decreasing tone in a spastic limb through sensory rhizotomies. Different treatment modalities have been introduced over years to address the complications of spasticity in CP children.

Cerebral palsy (CP) should not be considered as a diagnosis but as a label [2]; it is an umbrella term. The definition is not sufficiently precise to guarantee agreement as to which patients to include under this label, but the additional inclusion criteria required are not yet internationally standardized. It is a group of permanent disorders of the development of movement and posture, causing activity limitation, that are attributed to nonprogressive disturbances that occurred in the developing fetal or infant brain.

2. Spasticity management

Cerebral palsy is a difficult condition for many reasons, not least of which is because there is no cure. This neurological condition is caused by brain damage that is irreversible. This does not mean, however, that there is no hope for children diagnosed with cerebral palsy. Spasticity is a common symptom of cerebral palsy. It is characterized by stiff muscles that are difficult to control. In fact, several existing therapies can make a big difference, and there are now numerous emerging treatments that are changing how both children and adults live with cerebral palsy.

2.1 Physical therapy

Physical therapy relieves pain and muscle stiffness, improves mobility, and prevents future problems such as muscle tightness. It is always recommended as the first therapy intervention. It improves motor skills and can stop movement problems from worsening in the future. It includes varieties of treatment modalities such as strength, flexibility exercises, heat treatment, massages, and special equipment for CP children to give them more independence. How much the PT will help to improve the child's condition depends on the severity and CP type the child has. Mild cases only require some physical therapy. The best chance to improve the child's condition is with early intervention. Mobility can be improved by preventing contractures and joint dislocations by keeping the body strong and flexible. PT can improve the level of self-reliance of most CP children. The goal of PT is to make everyday movements easier. It can improve coordination, balance, strength, flexibility, endurance, pain management, posture, gait, and overall health.

The benefits of PT depend on the CP type:

- **Spastic**—It decreases the muscle tension and jerky movements.
- **Athetoid**—It increases muscle tone and gains more movement control.
- **Ataxic**—It improves balance problems.

The treatment plan will be based on the CP type. The child might have either hemiplegia, diplegia, or quadriplegia. Therapists design specific exercises and routines for each type, which helps the child regain movement in the affected area over time.

Other conditions such as scoliosis, thoracic kyphosis, lumbar lordosis, pelvic inclination, pelvic rotation, pelvic obliquity, knee deformity, shortened Achilles tendon, and hand and wrist deformities can be treated by PT. After the initial evaluation by the therapist, a treatment plan will be created, which might include a combination of exercises, muscle relaxing techniques, and special equipment to improve movement.

CP child either will have muscle hypotonia or hypertonia. Flexibility exercises and massages are usually used for the hypertonic child, which will develop mobility and prevent painful muscle tightening, which could require surgical intervention. On the other hand, the athetoid child will require strength training exercises to increase their muscle tone. Walking, posture, transitional movements, and sensory impairments such as touch and balance can be improved by certain exercises. Exercises that improve sitting, kneeling, and standing can improve posture. Infants use transitional movements to be able to walk, roll over, and sit up are examples of those movements.

Different mobility aids are to be used to make therapy more effective. Different orthotics equipment can be used to help with walking, posture, and joint mobility; braces, casts, splints, and shoe inserts are some examples. There are other tools that have been used in PT include exercise balls, resistance bands, free weights, swimming pools, hot and cold packs, and electric muscle stimulation (it improves gait and upper limb function).

As the child gets older, the physical therapist will change the program to meet the child's needs. Toddlers and the early school years are the most important stages of a child's life.

- **Toddlers**—Playtime is the main therapy focus during this stage. In this stage, children learn and gain experience through play, making it an essential part of early therapy. A therapist can help in certain areas such as overcoming toddlers' hesitancy to touch their faces or practicing certain movements that are necessary for learning and physical development.

- **Young children**—School-age children between 5 and 12 experience new movement issues because their bodies are growing. Physical therapy can ensure children to grow in a way that is matching to their motor function. At this stage, therapy will rely on exercises and orthotics. Instilling healthy habits and a proactive mindset is another goal at this stage.

Outcome of the therapy can be evaluated by observation and a set of standardized tests to measure motor function. Therapists will be looking for specific postures and movements that could be corrected to develop a strong treatment plan.

2.2 Occupational therapy

Health care providers usually recommend OT along with PT for CP children to provide easier independent lives because it has many benefits. On one hand, PT improves muscle tone and balance, and on the other hand, OT is helping children to accomplish daily living activities. According to the American Occupational Therapy Association (AOTA), OT helps people of all ages to learn how to improve their abilities to do their everyday activities [3]. Everyday school tasks, eating and drinking, dressing, hygiene, and other tasks necessary for daily use can be assisted by OT. Children with visual impairment, regardless of severity, can do their daily tasks by doing OT. Also, sensory-perceptual-motor (SPM) training, which helps to stimulate the senses of performing daily tasks more easily, can be assisted by OT. An occupational therapist usually uses visual input tools and cues, as well as verbal directions to help children in carrying out necessary everyday tasks. A cognitively impaired child can benefit from OT. Establishing daily schedules or routines to help those children some daily tasks such as remembering to dress, brush their teeth, and other tasks are needed to carry out their day.

The real challenge for CP children is their motor impairment, which makes their daily tasks difficult. For example, most children have difficulties with daily hygiene, moving around, posture, and completing school tasks due to their movement limitations. The occupational therapist will assess every child's needs individually to design a program to meet their personal goals. The main line of OT program includes stretching and guide motor output techniques and constraint-induced movement therapy (CIMT), which helps hemiplegic CP children [4], and neuromuscular facilitation techniques.

OT can help in other areas such as grasping objects; using computer and other electronics; opening doors; writing, holding, and reading books; playing; interacting with peers, caregivers, and parents; school and/or daycare activities; and sitting and standing up from tables and school desks. CP Children and their parents and caregivers can benefit from OT by watching children thrive both physically and emotionally. This progress reduces parents' stress and provides a sense of peace as the child becomes more independent and productive.

OT can take place in different settings such as outpatient offices, inpatient medical centers, at home, nursing centers, and OT providers. To obtain quality OT, the child must be under the care and supervision of a trained and licensed occupational therapist. By evaluating the child and assessing the child's strengths and weaknesses, they will be able to formulate an individualized plan to help the child best reach his or her goals. Per AOTA, licensed occupational therapists, besides they are licensed in their state to practice occupational therapy, have another degree in Social Services, Health, Biology, Chemistry, Psychology, Sociology, Human Development, and Anatomy & Physiology. To obtain their license, they must be graduated from an accredited school, do fieldwork hours, and pass the National Board for Certification in Occupational Therapy examination. The therapist will conduct a comprehensive assessment including testing the child's: motor skills, developmental condition, cognitive development and functioning, psychological needs, emotional needs, and home and school environment to be able to create an individualized treatment plan.

2.3 Oral medications

Oral medications have been used to decrease spasticity; however, they have a lot of side effects such as drowsiness, sedation, confusion, and fatigue. Benzodiazepines, like diazepam, are rarely used because of their strong sedating effects. They result in enhanced presynaptic inhibition, but because they are presumed to enhance the postsynaptic effects of GABA, they can only work if the GABA-mediated process functions. Benzodiazepines have a long half-life and an active metabolite. Benzodiazepine therapy is indicated in spinal cord injury and multiple sclerosis with possible application in traumatic brain injury, cerebral palsy, and cerebrovascular accident. Clinical effects include sedation and reduced anxiety, decreased resistance to passive range of motion, decreased hyperreflexia, and reduction in painful spasms. Side effects of all benzodiazepines include sedation, weakness, hypotension, gastrointestinal symptoms, memory impairment, incoordination, confusion, depression, and ataxia. Also, benzodiazepines are controlled substances with the potential for dependency. Diazepam is the most widely used benzodiazepine for spasticity management. The recommended initial dose is 2 mg 3 times daily with a maximum dose of 60 mg daily (20 mg 3 times daily). If nocturnal spasticity is the presenting problem, the patient should be started with a single dose at night.

Like benzodiazepines, baclofen works centrally. Baclofen binds with GABA-B receptors on brain and spinal membranes, restricting calcium influx into presynaptic nerve terminals, thereby reducing spasticity. The use of baclofen is indicated when spasticity is of spinal origin. The clinical effects include decreased resistance to passive range of motion, decrease in hyperreflexia, and reduction in painful spasms and clonus. Unlike benzodiazepines and baclofen, dantrolene sodium works peripherally at the level of the muscle fiber. It has no effect on neuromuscular transmission, but works by acting directly on the skeletal muscle, hindering the release of calcium from the sarcoplasmic reticulum, thereby preventing the excitation-contraction coupling mechanism. This affects both intrafusal and extrafusal fibers by decreasing the force of muscle contraction. However, this mechanism is not selective for muscles with increased tone, and the resulting generalized muscle weakness may weaken respiratory muscles. The use of dantrolene sodium is indicated in treating spasticity secondary to cerebrovascular accident and cerebral palsy, and has possible applications for traumatic brain injury, spinal cord injury, and multiple sclerosis. Clinical effects of dantrolene sodium include decreased resistance to passive range of motion, decrease in hyperreflexia and tone, and reduction in spasms and clonus. Another group of oral medications used in spasticity management includes clonidine and tizanidine, which are alpha 2 noradrenergic receptor agonists that release excitatory neurotransmitters and inhibit supraspinal facilitatory pathways [5].

Tizanidine is a new oral anti-spasticity agent that is selective in decreasing tone and spasm frequency in only spastic muscles, eliminating the unwanted side effect of generalized muscle weakness. Tizanidine is reported to have reduced symptoms of spasticity in patients with multiple sclerosis or spinal cord injury and is well tolerated in most patients. It is an imidazoline derivative like clonidine but without the cardiovascular effects when appropriately titrated. Tizanidine results in a direct reduction of excitatory amino acid release from spinal interneurons and inhibits facilitatory cerebrospinal pathways. Its peak effect occurs 1–2 hours following administration and its half-life is 2.5 hours. The clinical effects of tizanidine include reduced muscle tone, spasm frequency, and hyperreflexia. Animal studies with tizanidine demonstrate antinociceptive activity under specific conditions with increased dose titration [6].

As with other anti-spasticity medications, the potential side effects of tizanidine are dose-related and may be mitigated by dosage titration. The potential side effects include drowsiness, dry mouth, and dizziness. Literature suggests that tizanidine may be better tolerated than other anti-spasticity agents as measured by the global tolerance rating scale. In placebo-controlled studies, tizanidine has been shown to be effective in multiple sclerosis and spinal cord injury. It is also useful for spasticity of spinal pathology when weakness is of concern. Tizanidine may also prove effective in managing spasticity of cerebral origin.

Secondary oral and systemic agents include tiagabine, cyproheptadine, clonidine, lamotrigine, gabapentin, and carbidopa-levodopa [7]. Multiple medications have been recommended, of which the most recent addition is gabapentin.

The use of antihypertensive pharmacologic agents in treating spasticity is unclear because randomized trials have not been performed. Nifedipine has been used in a bit-and-swallow technique; more recently, captopril also has been found to be of benefit [8].

Anticholinergic medications are used in CP patients for different issues, such as uncontrollable limb and facial movements, muscle spasms, tremors, and excessive drooling. Anticholinergics block the area of the brain that causes muscle movement [9], which in turn helps to control many of the most common symptoms in CP children. Small doses of anticholinergic medications could be beneficial in some children, whereas other children will require higher dosages. The most common anticholinergics used in CP children include Robinul, Sinemet, benztropine mesylate, and trihexyphenidyl hydrochloride.

Antidepressant medications have been used to improve moods and enhance well-being. These types of drugs are not for everyone, and they have been used in children with depression, anxiety, and other mental and emotional problems that can come from living with a debilitating disorder. Antidepressants are generally used in combination with behavioral therapy [10]. Different antidepressants could be used, but the most commonly have been used are Celexa, Paxil, Prozac, Cymbalta, Lexapro, and Zoloft. Its side effects may differ from patient to patient. Different pain medications have been used, and the most commonly used ones are to control pain by reducing inflammation. Some CP children will experience chronic, long-term pain and anti-inflammatory medicine can be prescribed to relieve their pain. The most common types of anti-inflammatories prescribed to CP patients include nonsteroidal anti-inflammatory drugs (NSAIDs) and steroids. Some parents would rather use natural medications as opposed to traditional drugs, whereas others may try alternatives when the first line of prescribed medications fails to relieve symptoms. Others use a combination of complementary and alternative with conventional medicines. Complementary and alternative medications generally include biologically based supplements, homeopathic medicines, and herbal medicines.

2.4 Speech therapy

Health care providers will recommend speech therapy if the child has communication, swallowing, and breathing issues. Speech therapy provides a wide range of exercises to help children better communicate, address, and help in other disorders affecting speech. A child might have mild to severe speech impairment. However, a study from the National Institute of Neurological Disorders and Stroke (NIH) stated that despite not every CP child had speech impairment, many CP children had some form of speech impairment [11]. A licensed speech therapist evaluates every child to create the optimal individualized plan to help children have better communication. They provide exercises that help children understand gestures, words, numbers, sounds, and more. Also, they help with common problems for CP children such as breathing, swallowing, and digestion issues. They use a variety of exercises such as sign language, communication through writing and painting, winking, voice synthesizers, picture boards, and using augmentative communication devices. Theos' exercises will improve disorders such as pronunciation skills, vocabulary, development, listening skills, comprehension and formation of words, fluency, direct conversation engagement, and mouth and throat issues. The speech therapist will evaluate every child fully to come up with an individualized based on the child's needs. Dysphagia is a very common problem in CP children, which is secondary to physiological and neurological disorders, as well as irregularities in the throat. Choking on food and drinks, breathing difficulties, excessive coughing, and pulmonary aspiration of food and fluids must be addressed. Other associated conditions such as stuttering, dysphagia, aphasia, dyspraxia, intonation and rhythm issues, vocal tract problems, and dysarthria must be addressed too. Prevention and reduction ofother associated disorders such as easily choking on foods/liquids, extreme coughing, pulmonary aspiration, difficulties with breathing and dehydration, and malnutrition (typically because of choking on foods/liquids) also have to be one of the therapist's goals.

Communication is an important human experience, it shapes people's personalities. Children with communication issues are already at a disadvantage. Proper speech therapy helps the child to overcome their problems and let them communicate better. It will provide the child with the proper ways of communication and help him/her throughout the course of life, including daily living and social activities [12]. It provides other benefits such as learning, the ability to participate fully in school and home activities, better relationship development with friends, peers, and family, better socialization skills, and the ability to communicate ideas consistently and effectively. A master's degree in speech and language pathology is required to be a speech therapist/speech pathologist, and most states require that they get certified through the American Speech-Language-Hearing Association (ASHA). To obtain ASHA certification, speech pathologists must complete numerous courses dealing with the throat, mouth, speech, psychology, social work, and more [13].

2.5 Massage therapy

CP children can gain mental, emotional, and physical benefits from massage therapy. Massage therapy must be approved by the child's doctor before starting such a program. Massage therapy supports the treatment of body's connective tissues and muscles are massaged and stimulated through direct contact by a massage therapist to help healing and well-being of the patient. Direct hand pressure by the therapist will be applied to different body parts. The pressure could be light to heavy, depending on which body part is being stimulated. Therapists can use different types of massage techniques, which are more than 180 techniques with their hands, elbows, arms, and more.

Although the National Institutes of Health (NIH) states that more research is needed before recommending massage therapy to every CP child [14], the American Therapy Massage Association (AMTA) states that anyone can benefit from massage [15]. A published study by the University of Washington and Seattle Children's Hospital, and Integrative Touch for Kids, showed lessening of painful symptoms by using massage therapy. The study stated, "It is well documented that massage increases blood flow to the tissues and that enhanced blood flow encourages growth of new tissue and healing of wounds" [16].

Massage could stimulate the brain's pressure receptors when the cranium is massaged and stimulated, it gives a sense of calmness and in return, and the child will be able to focus and concentrate better. Fine and gross motor functioning improves when muscles are relaxed and less rigid. This helps all aspects of CP children's lives, including playing, socializing, learning, and carrying out daily tasks. Circulation and digestion issues are very common in the CP children. Immobility is the reason for circulation problems; on the other hand, the central and peripheral nervous system structural abnormalities might lead to digestion issues. Relieve tension in the abdominal muscles can help to improve digestion by reducing gassiness and bloating, stimulating peristalsis leading to better digestion, aiding in the release of digestive enzymes, and stimulating kidney and liver activity.

Improving sleep in CP children and adults can be achieved by massage therapy. According to the American Massage Therapy Association (AMTA) and a study published by the National Institutes of Health (NIH), massaging has an essential role in the quality of CP children's sleep (American Massage Therapy Association | AMTA) [17]".

Skin, exocrine glands, hair, and nails are the integumentary system of the body's organ that acts as the first line of defense against outside factors. Skin infections and other integumentary system problems are common in CP children because they cannot care for themselves. This system can be protected by stimulating the skin, improving skin tone and texture, assisting in body temperature regulation, promoting tissue repair, moisturizing skin, removing dead skin, and stimulating sensory receptors.

Massage therapy can be done in physical therapy centers, private massage therapy clinics, hospitals, chiropractic centers, athletic clubs and sports centers, spas, at home, and health clinics. Although massage therapy has shown many benefits, in some instances, it is not advisable. Message therapy is not recommended if the child has muscle and/or joint inflammation, fever, acute infections, skin disorders, open sores, swollen lymph nodes, vaccinations within the past 72 hours, blood clots, diarrhea, osteoporosis, and varicose veins.

Massage therapists cannot give any medical advice regarding your child's disorder or any other medical issue, psychological counseling, diet or nutrition counseling, touch private parts of the child's body, perform any type of surgery, and provide skin or cosmetology services. Usually, massage therapy sessions are not covered by insurance, and you might have to pay out-of-pocket expenses.

2.6 Hippotherapy

Hippotherapy is using horses and equine equipment to help CP children to develop better physical, emotional, and neurological functioning. Health care providers usually recommend classical and traditional therapies such as PT and OT, which help to strengthen muscles, improve balance and flexibility, and help with everyday living tasks. On the other hand, hippotherapy can help CP children greatly. It started overseas in the sixties, but it came to the United States after the great benefits it produces. Cognitive ability, neuromuscular problems, physical strength, and a heightened sense of well-being can be improved by hippotherapy [18]. A horse's movements can be channeled by using equine equipment. Hippotherapy and therapeutic horseback riding are two different therapy modalities to gain different benefits. The gait, rhythm, repetition, and tempo of a horse's movements have been proven to help with: balance, posture, strength, control, visual cues, sensory, endurance, abnormal muscle tone, social skills, control of the body's extremities, core strength in the trunk, and self-esteem.

After the health care provider ensures that child mental and physical challenges could benefit from this form of therapy, he/she can recommend hippotherapy. Also, the health care provider and the therapist must agree that the child's associated disorders will not be affected negatively by the physical challenges of hippotherapy. Hippotherapy can started at any age and has no age limit. Insurance companies usually do not cover the therapy, and you may pay out of pocket for it. A full evaluation of the child's physical, emotional, and cognitive strength must be done by the therapist to determine if the child is ready for hippotherapy and if any modifications must be provided for the child while sitting on the horse. Safety issues, including how to correctly mount and dismount the horse (with assistance), horse equipment, and what to expect when the horse moves, must be explained by the therapist. After safety training is in place, assisting and monitoring the child during mounting the horse and during the horse's movements, and walking alongside the horse and child while helping modify the horse's movements must be done by the therapist to make sure the child is safe. Hippotherapy will help to build physical strength and endurance and improve the child's well-being and sense of self. The sessions usually take place in horse farms created as specialized training areas. Physical therapists, speech therapists, or occupational therapists can provide the therapy sessions. They must go through extensive hippotherapy training (at least 3 years of their own field of study and 100 hours of hippotherapy training) and have their own certifications. Therapists need to have the following: They must learn in-depth knowledge of horse movement, how to handle emergencies, safety practices, the physical characteristics of horses, the association between human and horse movement and how to choose the appropriate exercises for each child's individual needs, and more. If the child's doctor approved the therapy, the therapist has ruled out any conditions that would prevent participation by the therapist.

2.7 Aquatic therapy

Aqua therapy or aquatic therapy is a group of water-based exercises improving a person's physical abilities and functions. The medical community recommended it as a way to help heal the body [19]. Aquatic therapy has shown improvement in CP children because by allowing them to move freely without putting stress or much weight on their bodies. Water is known to reduce weight by 90%.

Aquatic therapists help CP children to develop more muscle control, increase self-confidence, improve strength and physical function, and gain more life independence. The therapy itself has many physical and mental benefits to CP children. Physical benefits include improved heart function, increased resistance, relief and reduced pain in the joints and muscles, help in protecting against injuries, and reduced discomfort while exercising, help in building muscle and muscle control and better circulation, and improved endurance and flexibility. Mental and emotional benefits include improved confidence, better quality of life, strengthened socialization skills, improved sensory integration, and improved sense of independence.

The severity of the child's disorder, age, physical fitness level, and any associated illnesses or disorders will determine the best therapy program for the child. Popular aqua therapy exercises include swimming (at all levels, including learning to swim), aquatic yoga, water-based range of motion exercises, balance exercises *via* flotation devices in deep water, breath control exercises, assisted walking exercises, deep-water walk, and social games to help improve social interaction, eye contact, and sportsmanship. Flotation devices, toys, weights, compression vests, and balls are different equipment used during the aqua therapy session.

Children's safety is of utmost importance during the aqua sessions. In turn, most pools are generally smaller than standard-size pools and come with fiberglass or stainless-steel shells, built-in attached equipment, safety rails and ladders, thermostat to warm water, and easy-to-grip edges. An active AEA Aquatic Fitness Professional Certification (AFPC) is a requirement for any physical or occupational therapist to carry out the sessions. The session lasts 30 to 45 minutes depending on the child's individual needs. Kids must bring swimsuits, towels, and water shoes to each session. Some classes may provide these items depending on the program and the family's financial status.

2.8 Osteopathic manipulation

A trained osteopathic doctor (DO) can provide osteopathic manipulation therapy (OMT) by applying a gentle manipulation of the musculoskeletal system to relieve symptoms and improve overall wellness in patients. The philosophy used by DOs is a holistic, preventative approach with a focus on the musculoskeletal system, how it is linked to disease, and how it can be manipulated for treatment. Despite there being some evidence that OMT can help CP children move better and feel better, the studies are small and have mixed results on how OMT can help those children.

OMT is based on the notion that all body systems are connected, and this connection affects disease and wellness [20]. Osteopathic manipulation therapy is based on a hands-on approach, which is an important part of OMT. DOs use stretching and gentle pressure to manipulate joints and muscles. Musculoskeletal disorders such as back and neck pain or sports-related injuries are common examples of OMT. Some DOs use the technique for different types of conditions, citing a healing touch as crucial to wellness.

OMT has been used as an alternative therapy for CP children complaining of musculoskeletal system symptoms. It is a complementary therapy to more traditional therapies such as PT, OT, surgery, and pain medication to relieve symptoms and pain, improve mobility and reduce spasticity, and more. Cranial osteopathy can be applied to the head and neck. It is a subtle gentle manipulation of the skull that can be used in babies but that can also be used in children and adults.

OMT was studied to see its usefulness in 55 spastic CP children (moderate to severe spasticity) between 20 months and 12 years of age [21]. There were three groups: a control group with no treatment, a group that received acupuncture, and a group that received cranial osteopathic manipulation along with myofascial release. Eleven outcomes were listed as outcomes. The acupuncture group had no significant positive outcomes; on the other hand, the cranial osteopathy group had a positive outcome in two measures (total Gross Motor Function Measurement and the mobility part of the Functional Independence Measure for Children) in comparison with the control group. In another study, thirteen children diagnosed with both cerebral palsy and chronic constipation were studied using OMT. Children were divided into two groups; one group received OMT, while the other group received OMT and traditional medical treatment for constipation. At the conclusion of the study, both groups had equally positive benefits and improvements in constipation [22].

A larger recent study of the use of cranial manipulation in CP children has cast doubt over the treatment's effectiveness. A British study for 6 months of 142 children using cranial osteopathy. There were two equal numbers of children in each group, and one group received the treatment, while the second group was placed in a control group. The children's movement was evaluated after 6 months, and there were no statistically significant improvements as compared to the children from the control group [23]. Children's parents in the treatment group felt that their children had positive gains, in comparison with only a few parents in the control group. Reported positive results by the parents were better sleep, better use of arms and legs, and improved mood [24]. It is not clear if OMT may or may not help CP children, it is different from child to child how it helps. If the therapy is administered by a licensed DO, there is almost no risk of side effects or complications with this type of therapy.

2.9 Chiropractic care

Chiropractic care is a natural type of treatment, which helps several musculoskeletal and nervous system conditions. It is conducted by licensed chiropractors performing different techniques to help reduce pain and spasms and restore proper nervous system function. According to the American Chiropractic Association (ACA), the focus of chiropractic care is the musculoskeletal system disorders and nervous system disorders [25]. The Palmer College of Chiropractic reports that "*no part of your body escapes the dominance of your nervous system*" [26]. Poor health and improper nervous system functioning could be because of misalignment or other improper functions of the spinal cord and other areas of the body. Treatment focuses on different body parts, like the back, neck, shoulders, hands, and joints in the arms and legs. Despite chiropractors can prescribe certain medications if needed, no medications have been used in the treatment.

Some studies showed neuromuscular and mobility improvement in CP children by using chiropractic care. Some were able to sit up (when they previously could not), walk upstairs without assistance, and use their arms and hands better. Reduction in: Pain and muscle stiffness, breathing problems, drooling, muscle contractions, neck pain, musculoskeletal conditions, gait issues, spine issues, anxiety and stress, headaches and chest pain, leg/arm problems, speech problems due to respiratory issues, spasticity, and urinary incontinence were the improved areas after chiropractic care.

After taking a full medical history, the chiropractor will ask you and/or your child specific questions about pain and any activities that make the pain worse [27]. A physical exam must be done (which could include diagnostic tests such as X-rays or an MRI). The following areas could be studied: neurological integrity, range of motion, muscle tone and strength, abnormalities, misalignment, and flexion-distraction therapy. Treatment will be designed based on the child's medical history and physical exam results. The most common forms of treatment include spine adjustments, which can include low spine adjustments, full spine adjustments, the "Activator" technique, and/or the "Gonstead" technique, adjustment to joint dysfunctions, massaging, electrical stimulation, traction, heat/cold applications, and myofascial release. Treatment sessions usually are 30 minutes to an hour, depending on the chiropractor's techniques and the child or family's concerns or medical issues. For example, lower back pain treatment may require 1–3 visits per week for up to 2–3 months. Sessions could be conducted in hospitals, clinics, or a private provider's office. Most chiropractors have their own private offices.

Children and parents could get scared during sessions by some maneuvers. Adjustment by the chiropractor could make a popping sound, this does not mean that any bones are broken, and it is from releasing gas from fluids surrounding the joints. Mild discomfort by the child or if the child cries (due to pain) or complains the procedures are too painful, please discuss your concerns with the chiropractor. Chiropractor care usually is not painful. It is very important to choose a well-trained chiropractor by considering his education, training, licensing, and experience working with other healthcare providers and easily coordinating care. The treatment is considered "complementary" care, and it might be not covered by insurance.

2.10 Homeopathy treatment

It can be used to relieve CP children's difficult symptoms such as relieving pain, improving mobility, and relieving many of the associated symptoms and conditions of CP. Homeopathy is a complete integrated medical system, a complete theory of medical practice that considers a complementary, or alternative, treatment to Western medicine [28]. Homeopathy is a modern alternative medicine like the traditional Chinese medicine, which has evolved over thousands of years. There is a lot of criticism for homeopathy, but many people are claiming it has helped relieve their symptoms. Almost, there are no risks of working with a trained homeopath.

Samuel Hahnemann, a German who created the homeopathy in the 1700s based on the idea that with a little prompting, the body has a remarkable capacity to heal itself. The name homeopathy came from the Greek words "homosis" meaning similar and "pathos" meaning suffering. Homeopathy has two main principles. The first is the idea that like cures like. When a person suffers from a certain symptom, if a substance is triggering that symptom was given to that person, this substance will cure it rather than make it worse. The main idea behind this belief is that the substance will enhance the body's natural ability to fight the illness or symptom. The second principle is that the treating substance must be given only in very small, dilute amounts, which is thought to be sufficient to trigger.

Remedies extracted from origin such as plants and minerals have been given to patients to treat symptoms and illnesses. Some are toxic and poisonous, like arsenic and belladonna, but others are benign, and all are made with extremely minute amounts of the active ingredient. Some remedies' formulation has a very low concentration of the active ingredient to be considered chemically insignificant. They come in pill or solution form, and they are over the counter and are regulated by the U.S. Food and Drug Administration.

Some CP children's symptoms can be relieved by homeopathy; for example, seizure control was described in an article published by the journal, The American Homeopath. Two children failed their anticonvulsant medicines and tried homeopathy to help control their seizures. One boy has severe CP was crippled by seizures and used a variety of over-the-counter remedies for 3 months, and his seizure severity was reduced first and then the frequency. The other case was a severe CP girl and seizures. Homeopathic remedies were used for just over a year. Eight years later she was still seizure-free [29]. A seven-year-old CP boy who was mostly immobile, blind, and incontinent was described in another study. He was on homeopathic treatment for 2 months; he has improvement in his mobility, also he has improvement in his hair lose, became mobile with the help of PT. Other studies have shown either more limited or no results from using homeopathy to treat CP children.

Because the treatment is highly individualized, studying homeopathy is very difficult. Treatment methodology does not allow giving the same remedies to a big group of children having the same symptoms. Many symptoms can be treated with homeopathy. These include mobility, muscle weakness, spasticity, joint pain, digestive issues, and associated conditions (asthma, anxiety, and skin). Homeopathic medicines are safe because they are FDA regulated. There is a strong belief among scientists that remedies have in role in curing or relieving any symptoms because of the very low doses of substances used. Others believe homeopathy has a placebo effect and makes people feel better.

Sessions must be conducting by a trained and certified homeopathic practitioner even there are very limited risks of using homeopathy. Before using homeopathic for your child, you should ask your doctor if there are any reasons you should not try homeopathy. There is a rare risk of side effects or interaction with another medication by using a small amount of active ingredient. Homeopathy has some criticism but also has its supporters. Despite there are limited large-scale studies that prove its efficacy, there are a plenty of case studies. There is plenty of anecdotal evidence and studies showed the benefits to the patients by using this therapy. If your CP child failed the conventional treatments, you might consider consulting a trained homeopathic practitioner.

2.11 Pet therapy

Pet therapy, or animal-assisted therapy, is a complementary therapy for CP children to obtain a lot of benefits from PT and other types of treatment. Working with animals can help CP children reach their goals when added to classic therapies. It is of great importance to work with therapists and animals that are trained and licensed and have experience working with CP children. Pet therapy is the use of well-trained animals to promote wellness, boost mood, and help therapy, and other broad uses in mental and physical health care [30]. There are different ways of pet therapy, either informal or formal. When a trained dog visits a nursing home or hospital to cheer up residents and patients, it is informal. On the other hand, when the animal is the central aid or participant in a guided therapy session, it is formal. Dogs are frequently used in pet therapy but other kinds of animals like cats, horses, and even guinea pigs can be involved.

A study published by the U.S. National Institutes of Health showed that "personal and social benefits gained by dog-assisted therapy may aid in the prevention, improvement, and development of children with various disabilities" [31]. Pet therapy has been used in different situations such as chemotherapy sessions, dental work, and other potentially scary or stressful procedures for children, or even adults, PT sessions to treat injury or a stroke, mental health problems, or for residents in long-term care facilities. It is also commonly used to assist CP children with disabilities.

There are documented benefits of working with animals with special needs of children and adults in formal and informal settings. In mental health cases, being around animals and interacting with them have been shown to lower anxiety, increase relaxation, reduce loneliness, provide comfort, and increase mental stimulation [32]. Physical benefits of working with animals have been well documented, including lowering blood pressure and heart rate, improving cardiovascular health, and reducing pain. Petting and playing with animals have been shown to increase serotonin and reduce cortisol, which together promote less stress in the body.

Having an animal in the PT session for CP children can provide numerous benefits like working with animals during PT helps children reach specific goals, sessions will be less stressful, and children are more engaged and enthusiastic about doing the work. Animals provide good physical support to the children to do their exercises, children prefer using animals than an object for support, and animals motivate children to work harder, meet their goals, and return for subsequent sessions. CP children usually have a lot of mental health issues and behavioral challenges such as ADHD, depression, and anxiety as comorbid conditions. Animals can help improve children's mood, reduce anxiety, and reduce stress. Benefits of behavioral therapy sessions using animals are motivation, support, encouragement, and someone to bond with and help a child be more engaged and enthusiastic about treatment [33].

One study established a goal for disabled CP children therapy using trained dogs to assist. Results have shown that before therapy children were unable to complete the therapy sessions, but all completed the animal sessions and met their goals after therapy. The animals helped them break down resistance and fear and to carry on with successful therapy sessions.

Children showed improvement in their communication and became better able to tell others what they need or want. They became more sympathetic from working with dogs and they became better able to ask for help and provide help to others. Also, their social skills have improved. Dogs are the most used animals because of how easy they are to be trained and their love of people, but other animals can be trained to work with children with special needs as well. Equine therapy and dolphin therapy have been used as well. Equine therapy may include riding, petting, or caring for horses. The outcome of the sessions relay on the child's goals but working with horses has the added benefits of getting children outside and improving self-confidence. There are additional potential benefits from the dolphin therapy beside the obtained benefits from other kinds of animals, but it is not common. CP children with mobility issues and pain can be easier to work in the water. However, dolphin therapy is relatively new, and there is little available evidence that it helps. This therapy is expensive but there is an increase in the number of facilities offering this therapy. You should work only with a trained and licensed therapist.

Informal therapy can help CP children who may have to spend time in the hospital for treatments, surgery, and for recovery after surgery by making them more relaxed in a stressful environment. They provide comfort, reduce anxiety, make the hospital setting feel more like home, and offer a feeling of love and acceptance for children who are struggling. Also, children can communicate with and relate better to doctors and nurses. Pet therapy can be a great way for CP children and other disabilities to get more out of their therapy sessions **3.1.**

2.12 Pilates

A fully integrated program of exercises using special apparatus, amid to improve physical strength, flexibility, posture, endurance, and mental awareness. It is easy to be used for beginners, they can use it because it does not require heavy weights or strenuous cardiovascular work, it is easy on the joints, and it has many health and fitness benefits. It can be used by all ability levels and can provide a significant strength workout for advanced athletes or a gentler workout for beginners, patients recovering from injury, or those with physical limitations. For CP children and adults, exercise of any type may seem daunting. Physical activity and supervised exercise have many benefits for CP patients as well as healthy people. Pilates is a suitable program to be adopted by people with physical limitations and to improve the CP symptoms while also increasing mobility and range of motion.

Pilates became very popular in the modern area, but it is nearly 100 years old, and it was created by Joseph Pilates in the 1920s. It involves the use of low-impact movements that focus on muscle strength, flexibility, and endurance [33]. Good posture and spinal alignment, balance between muscles, and core strength are the focus. Many moves can be done without equipment, but Pilates machines are used to help do specific movements and exercises.

Physical activity of any type is beneficial for everyone. If workouts routine is created to match an individual's ability level and limitations, any type of exercise improves cardiovascular health, muscle strength, bone density, and other areas of the body and mind. Great health benefits can be obtained by Pilates, such as greater flexibility, improved balance and posture, reduced back pain, greater strength and stability in the core, improved overall muscle strength, greater muscle endurance, and better mental well-being.

Symptoms of adults and children can be improved by practicing Pilates, but other specific benefits are to be achieved. A child may have trouble to control his muscle movements, and he/she might be able to bend or straighten his/her leg but nothing in between. Guided work on a reformer (Pilates equipment with a sliding frame) could help children develop greater control over their movements. Those exercises can be done while the child is lying down, often in a more comfortable position.

Targeting children's trunks with physical and strength training could significantly improve mobility and balance, a study showed. Children, before the study started, were not able to sit up by themselves. They were trained using specialized equipment used to target their trunk muscles and hip joints. After several weeks of training, they were better able to control movements and could sit and balance independently. The study did not use Pilates movements, but other studies have demonstrated that Pilates training can improve strength and posture stability in the trunk. Children who used Pilates have the chance to improve their stability, so they are able to sit up much easier, be more stable and balanced, and have greater control over their movements.

There is plenty of anecdotal evidence from personal stories that practicing Pilates can benefit adults and children with physical limitations. Gaining greater strength, posture, and balance between muscles that were previously weaker or stronger than others was described by adults. Stories of children who used Pilates movements in their PT sessions made them more independent, have greater joint range of motion, and have greater muscle strength that was once weak and difficult to control. The improvements in strength, balance, flexibility, and posture all help reduce pain as well [34].

Emotional and mental benefits of using Pilates can be experienced by children. The improvements in a child's pain and movement using Pilates could be great, and they give a great sense of control, achievement, and even relaxation with less stress. A positive body image can be achieved in all types of people, better with and without disabilities by using Pilates. It is recommended to try Pilates under the supervision of a trained instructor. The movements are generally easy, but it is easy to be done incorrectly. Most of the poses and movements are very specific and it could be of benefit if supervised by a trainer to correct and guide them, especially in CP children. Hospitals, medical centers, and physical therapy centers offer in-house Pilates classes and other types of exercises, so start with your medical team to find out how you can safely get started with Pilates.

2.13 Yoga

Yoga is an ancient practice of mixing physical with spiritual elements. Despite it being old Indian practice, nowadays it became more popular than ever. Stress relief, flexibility, strength, and other health improvements can be achieved by practicing Yoga. It can also be of great help to CP children and adults.

There are few clinical studies on yoga's effect on CP children. However, benefits were greatly documented from individual stories, anecdotes, and case studies showing Yoga, specially modified for personal needs, can have a positive effect on CP patients' life quality. While some studies for CP children are inconclusive [35], but evidence that yoga provides health benefits, in general, has been documented. There are different branches of complete yoga practice, like breathing exercises and meditation, but recent practitioners focus on asana, the postures.

Asanas are specific positions that are held for sometimes and that are designed to prepare the body with strength and clarity for meditation. On the one hand, Asanas had classic and original purposes; in recent practice, they provide several physical and mental health benefits. On the other hand, hatha yoga is a series of poses that are held for a period of time with a focus on breathing.

Benefits such as weight loss and better eating habits have been shown in studies of people practicing yoga [36]. Ashtanga and Power Yoga are intense and strenuous, but other forms of Yoga are not. Stimulating metabolism while helping with weight loss and weight management can be achieved by practicing Yoga.

The mindfulness practiced during yoga also helps people eat more mindfully, eating smaller portions, and making better choices. Overall better physical fitness, improved cardiovascular health, and lower blood pressure are proven benefits of Yoga. Yoga like PT improves muscle strength, balance, gain mobility in CP children often modified for a person's needs, or limitations to help children see benefits. Yoga stretches the body and enhances flexibility, joints range of motion, and over mobility. Yoga especially can stretch the spine and help realign it better [37]. Spine stretching increases the spaces between vertebrae, which in turn decreases pressure on nerves. Less muscular tension and relaxation throughout the whole body is the overall result. Other less tangible benefits for CP children include relaxation, less stress, better body image, and an overall better sense of well-being.

Health care providers should consider Yoga as part of CP children and adults' treatment plans. Asana postures are not possible to be done as they are described in patients with any degree of physical disability. Only, they must be adapted for patient with a disability to see benefits. Chair yoga is a perfect example of adapted Yoga in CP patients allowing them to enjoy the benefits of Yoga while they are confined to a wheelchair. The positions are modified from the perspective of sitting in a chair like a child with a balance problem can still use a pose, but while sitting. Other yoga adaptations involve different other props, such as blocks or straps, and the help of a trained practitioner or coach who has experience working with disabled patients.

Asanas are the most common yoga type in the west, mindfulness is the most important part of this ancient practice. Yoga users must be mindful by focusing on the body's posture and breathing while performing the poses, active practice of meditation by sitting still and focusing on the present, most often by focusing on breathing while you are practicing yoga. Meditation can benefit CP children and adults by lowering stress and anxiety, reducing gastrointestinal symptoms, improving sleep, and reducing feelings of depression.

Trying yoga is a good way to see real and positive benefits in CP children. It is very important to work with a professional who is trained in instructing yoga positions and can work with people who have physical disabilities. The poses will need to be adapted and it takes an experienced professional to know how to adapt them to everyone. Despite yoga being an old practice, but nowadays it has been modified and adapted in ways that are varied and positive. Yoga can help CP children to be able to participate in an activity that helps them move better, feel better, and have a greater sense of self-confidence and control. The many benefits of yoga are why every child should give it a try.

2.14 Functional electrical stimulation

It is developed initially to use electrical pulses to stimulate muscles in patients suffering from paralysis. Functional electrical stimulation (FES) currently treating different disorders like CP. It has been tested in clinical trials, and it has been tested for different disorders such as stroke, multiple sclerosis, and CP. In CP children, it is shown to improve range of motion, muscle mass and strength, walking speed, spasticity, gait, and foot and ankle positioning. Still, more research is needed for CP children and other neuromuscular disorders.

FES is a simple technology of a small device that delivers an electrical impulse to a muscle. It is a low-energy current that acts like a tiny shock to activate nerves, which in turn causes the muscle to move [38]. It has been used in paralyzed muscles in a person after an accident who cannot move them. It helps a person with small-scale muscle movements like voiding the bladder and swallowing, as well as with larger movements such as walking, grasping objects, or standing up. Also, it has been used after stroke in a person who has lost some muscle function, and for those with neurological disorders or head injuries. The procedure is safe and not painful because the electrical energy delivered is low. The electrical impulse may cause a little tingling or, sometimes, a slight burning sensation. It is not considered as a lifelong mobility aid, but it is a functional treatment restoring function. Usually, its use is for a short-term to help retrain muscles and restore some degree of voluntary muscle function. Implanted electrical stimulation devices are a new technology helping paralyzed patients to restore some muscle movement.

Spastic CP is very common and accounts for about 70 and 80 percent of all children with CP [39]. Children have painful stiff muscles, and their reflexes are exaggerated. Spastic CP children have different degrees of trouble walking. Commonly, they have involuntary limb movement, continuous muscle spasms, joint contractures, and limited flexibility. Some studies demonstrated that spastic CP children have a better and easy walk by applying FES. In one study 32 children, with an average age of 10 years, received eight weeks of daily functional electrical stimulation to the muscles [40]. There were two groups, an FES group and a control group. Evaluation schedule was at the beginning of the study, eight weeks of treatment, and then six weeks after that. The study has an end point of assessing the children's ability to walk and their own perceptions of how they walked before. FES group children showed great improvements in how they perceived their ability to walk. They felt that they are walking better and with less pain.

In a hemiplegic spastic CP children study, FES improves gait abnormalities [41]. The children in the study were able to walk using braces. FES has replaced children's braces or splints. Evaluation was done before and after the treatment, toe-walking and other asymmetries were improved greatly, and all children were able to walk more symmetrically.

Foot drop; There is a common problem in CP children, they have trouble picking up their feet to take steps, and their toes drag while they are walking. They can overcome this by lifting their knee up higher or swinging it outward to be able to elevate the foot off the floor while walking. This can cause pain and other issues later by doing this awkward movement to keep the foot from dragging. Braces or orthotics can correct the foot drop at the expense of the child's movement limitation. On the other hand, FES shows great promise to treat foot drop in CP children. FES device was used in a group of children for 4 months, and they have gait evaluations periodically. They had no change in the speed of their walk, but there was improvement in their ankle flexion and foot with reduced awkward movements to avoid dragging the toes.

Despite the positive study results of using FES in CP children, still it is not accepted as a common treatment. Currently, enrolling in clinical trials is the only way to get the treatment. Using FES can give a child hope to move free from awkwardness and pain. While the treatment is not widely available, its apparent effectiveness and safety mean that its use will likely become more widespread.

2.15 Chemo-denervation

Chemo-denervation such as using botulinum toxin type A has proved easier, more effective, and less painful for patients. First clinically introduced in the United States in the early 1980s, botulinum toxin is a potent neurotoxin derived from the anaerobic bacteria *Clostridium botulinum*, but when used in treatment, no serious systemic toxin effects have been reported [42].

The medication is more costly than alcohol or phenol, but the cost is offset by less physician time and the lack of anesthesia. The formation of antibodies has been a concern, but this can be prevented by allowing 2 months to 3 months between injections. Botulinum toxin works by acting in the neuromuscular junction, preventing the release of acetylcholine, which results in functional denervation. It can be given without EMG and anesthesia, does not cause dysesthesias, and is no more painful than an injection of saline solution. Effects are local and last 3 months to 4 months or longer. It is contraindicated during pregnancy, lactation, in individuals with neuromuscular disorders (such as myasthenia gravis), in patients taking aminoglycosides, or in those who have a known allergy to the drug. Adverse effects are not common and are usually associated with the site of injection, such as bleeding, bruising, soreness or redness at the injection site, or diffusion to nearby muscle groups. In patients that do not respond to botulinum toxin, possible reasons should be considered before labeling the patient as unresponsive. Reasons could be related to injection technique, improper toxin storage, or the patient's individual characteristics. Overall, botulinum toxin has proven clinically to be effective, safe, and less painful than other invasive therapies [43].

Botulinum toxin is available in serotypes A and B, which have different unit potencies, side-effect profiles, and dilution schedules. Both have been used in children with cerebral palsy, although serotype A has been used more extensively. Dosing guidelines have been suggested for botulinum toxin A for adult and pediatric patients. Adult recommendations are available for botulinum toxin B, but studies are ongoing for pediatric patients [44].

Some results suggest that botulinum toxin type A can be effective in reducing muscle tone over a longer period, but not in preventing development of contractures in spastic muscles. Mechanical and functional alterations can arise from the muscle tissue itself even though the nervous system is the site of the primary lesion. The gross mechanical changes occur in skeletal muscle secondary to spasticity and during development of contracture. Muscle stiffness can change for a variety of structural reasons, only one of which is altered fiber length. There is currently no evidence in the literature that muscle fiber length is shortened in contracture or in spastic skeletal muscle. Contracture formation results from inappropriate architectural adaptation of extremity muscles in response to upper motor neuron lesion [45].

Several studies have reported the successful use of botulinum toxin A for the treatment of drooling in children with cerebral palsy, using injection into the submandibular or parotid glands alone or in combination with other agents. In some studies, the beneficial effects have lasted for up to 4 months without serious side effects or disturbances of oral function [46].

Other treatments include *chemical neurolysis*, in which the nerve conduction is impaired using chemical agents and therapeutic nerve block using phenol or alcohol. The goals of these treatments are to prevent muscle contractures and improve the patient's function. A common side effect is that after the nerve is injected, alcohol levels measure above the legal limit in children. Other side effects include damage to sensory and motor nerves, pain at injection site, scarring, and dysesthesias. To ensure the correct site, an injection must be made using an electrical stimulator [47].

2.16 Neurosurgical approaches

Another treatment used to alleviate spasticity in children with cerebral palsy is *rhizotomy*. Studies have shown that performing selective dorsal rhizotomy at a young age can reduce the need for orthopedic surgery [48]. Goals of rhizotomy are decreased tone, increased mobility, and the facilitation of care for the patient; however, the reduction in spasticity cannot be predicted and sometimes results in excessive hypotonia [49]. The procedure is very meticulous, requiring general anesthesia and a neurophysiologist who must be present to identify which nerve is to be severed.

Other *neurosurgical approaches* include peripheral neurectomy, myelotomy, and dorsal column electrical stimulation.

It has been established that oral baclofen does not cross the blood-brain barrier effectively and that higher doses of the medication result in serious side effects. Intrathecal baclofen results in a greater decrease in spasticity by allowing higher concentrations of baclofen in the cerebrospinal fluid at about 1% of the daily oral dosage [50].

To be considered for intrathecal baclofen pump placement, the patient must have severe lower limb spasticity that does not respond to other less-invasive treatments. The patient must first be given a trial of 50 μg baclofen through a lumbar puncture or spinal catheter. If unresponsive, 75 μg can be tried after 24 hours and a third trial of

100 μg can be tried 24 hours after that, after which if the patient is still unresponsive, he or she must be excluded from the treatment [51]. Implantation lasts 1–2 hours, and the pump is easy to refill subcutaneously. It is programmed by a computer-controlled radiotelemetry programmer that is linked to the pump's internal computer and selects the rate and pattern of baclofen administration. Complications to intrathecal baclofen include hypersensitivity to baclofen, intolerance to the side effects of baclofen including drug tolerance, cerebrospinal fluid leakage, pump pocket seroma, hematoma, infection, and soft tissue erosion. The objective of intrathecal baclofen is to individualize the patient's dose and infusion so that the lowest dose that yields the greatest response can be achieved [52]. In comparison, intrathecal baclofen has less complications and side effects than other treatments and more generalized results in both cerebral and spinal spasticity, making intrathecal baclofen the most effective current tool for the treatment of spasticity in non-ambulant individuals. A recent systematic review showed that there was no evidence to support the clinical use of intrathecal baclofen in ambulant individuals with hypertonicity without further rigorous longitudinal studies [17]. As a precaution, families are prescribed diazepam or diazepam rectal as well as oral baclofen to have at home. If there is evidence of withdrawal, one of these medications is administered, and the patient is instructed to go immediately to the emergency department. Although aggressive use of benzodiazepines and oral baclofen may be helpful, recognition, and return to appropriate intrathecal baclofen dosage are essential for rapid recovery [53].

2.17 Orthopedic procedures

Orthopedic procedures are the most frequently performed operations for spasticity. The targets of these operations are muscles, tendons, or bones. Muscles may be denervated and tendons and muscles may be released, lengthened, or transferred. The goals of surgery may include reducing spasticity, increasing range of motion, improving access for hygiene, improving the ability to tolerate braces, or reducing pain. Orthopedic problems that may result from a spastic limb include cubital or carpal tunnel syndrome, spontaneous fracture, dislocation of the hip or knee, and heterotopic ossification.

The most common orthopedic procedure for the treatment of spasticity is a *contracture release*. In this procedure, the tendon of a muscle that has a contracture is partially or completely cut. The joint is then positioned at a more normal angle, and a cast is applied. Regrowth of the tendon to a new length occurs over several weeks. Serial casting may be used to gradually extend the joint. Following cast removal, physical therapy is used to strengthen the muscles and improve range of motion.

Spastic muscles in the shoulder, elbow, forearm, hands, and legs may all be treated with tendon or muscle lengthening. Spasticity in the shoulder muscles may cause abduction or adduction and internal rotation of the shoulder. Abduction results in difficulties with balance, which then affects walking and transferring, and adduction causes problems when reaching for an object or with hygiene and personal care. An operation known as a slide procedure may be used to lengthen the supraspinatus muscle in an abducted spastic shoulder. With adducted shoulders, the surgeon can perform a release of all four muscles that typically cause this deformity.

In an operation known as a tendon transfer, the orthopedic surgeon moves a tendon from the spot at which it attaches to the spastic muscle. With the tendon transferred to a different site, the muscle can no longer pull the joint into a deformed position. In some situations, the transfer allows improved function. In others, the joint retains passive but not active function. Ankle-balancing procedures are among the most effective interventions.

The goal of surgical-orthopedic treatment, which is basically symptomatic, improve, or facilitate the movement to solve the functional or fixed contractures preventing further rehabilitation, to solve the deformation that reduces or prevents movement, sitting, causing pain as in the cases of hip luxation, or threaten respiration as in cases of severe scoliosis. Subluxation and dislocations of the hip in children with CP are most common in children and adolescents who do not walk. We must bear in mind the saying that every child and adolescent with CP has a hip disorder until proven otherwise. The occurrence of dislocation of the hips makes furniture, hygiene and often causes pain. Requires regular radiological studies to the hips once or twice a year during growth, to discover any hip dislocation at an early stage. Subluxation and luxation of the hips are treated surgically. The decision about surgery should bring those involved in the treatment of patients, carefully weighing hopper performs coarse benefits, and harms of surgery. Surgery is necessary to balance the muscle forces around the hip and normalize abnormal anatomic relationships [54].

Osteotomy and arthrodesis involve operations on the bones and are usually accompanied by operations to lengthen or split tendons to allow for fuller correction of the joint deformity. Osteotomy can be used to correct a deformity that cannot be fixed with other procedures. In an osteotomy, a small wedge is removed from a bone to allow it to be repositioned or reshaped. A cast is applied, while the bone heals in a more natural position. Osteotomy procedures are most used to correct hip displacements and foot deformities. Arthrodesis is a fusing together of bones that normally move independently. This fusion limits the ability of a spastic muscle to pull the joint into an abnormal position. Arthrodesis procedures are performed most often on the bones in the ankle and foot. In triple arthrodesis, the three joints of the foot are exposed, the cartilage is removed, and screws are inserted into the bones, fixing the joints into position. With a short walking cast in place for 6 weeks or until the bones have fully healed, the patient may bear weight immediately after the operation (http://wemove.org/spa/spa_oss.html, 2007).

The risks of developing a structural spinal deformity ranges from 24% to 36% for scoliosis and 50% for lordosis for an average of 4–11 years after selective dorsal rhizotomy [55].

Other principles include single event, multilevel surgery; surgery is delayed if possible (more than 6 years). Spasticity management is used as an adjunct to surgical intervention.

2.18 Intensive suit therapy

Intensive suit therapy is a new and experimental treatment for CP children helping them to improve muscle tone, posture, and movement. Despite more studies being needed to confirm its treatment effectiveness, some therapists offer it to their patients because they feel it is useful as a treatment option. It consists of an orthotic suit that includes a hat, knee pads, and specially designed therapeutic shoes. It also has rings that allow bungee cord-like ropes to be inserted and adjusted according to the child's height.

The child goes through a group of specific exercises in a therapeutic setting, and the suit brings the body into proper alignment and helps to improve abnormal muscle tone, while the suit is on and the elastic ropes are adjusted. Simply, it retrains the brain to recognize the new, corrected body movements. It reduces ataxia, spasticity, and other symptoms that are typically associated with cerebral palsy.

Different types of suits are available, and each one comes with a specific exercise program and training method, but all work in a similar therapeutic concept. The most common suits are Adeli Suit, NeuroSuit, Polish Suit, and TheraSuit. Some suits, such as the NeuroSuit and TheraSuit, offer elbow pads and gloves, which help to increase the function and strength of the arms. In1971, Russia's space program, the first suit was used, allowed cosmonauts to keep their normal muscle tone while in a weightless environment. In the late 1960s, the Penguin Suit was invented by the Russian Center for Aeronautical and Space Medicine, and it was reliable and fully functional in helping astronauts to prevent disabilities. In the early 1990s, a similar suit was invented by the Pediatric Institute of the Russian Academy of Medical Sciences for CP children and other neuromuscular disorders. This suit was patented in 1994 and became available for therapeutic use. Other suits were invented later for the same purpose.

School of Physical Therapy at the Pacific University reported some improvement in standing ability in the patients who underwent intensive suit therapy from their program [56]. The same conclusion came from a published study by the National Institutes of Health (NIH) [57]. More research is needed to understand the effectiveness of this therapy. Professor Siemionowa, who was member of the team that invented the "Adeli Suit," concluded that, after the second or third exercise session, children showed a decrease in their spasticity and diminished hyperkinesis in a study done by his institute. The conclusion of the stay was that the suit has a positive effect on the vestibular system, leading to improvements in balance and spatial awareness. The use of the intensive suit therapy in conjunction with the traditional therapy has proven to be the most beneficial effect. In research published in 2011 by the Online Journal of Health and Allied Sciences, 30 spastic diplegic CP children, ranging from ages 4 to 12 years, were studied by a team of physicians [14]. Children were in a combined program of traditional PT and intensive suit therapy for 2 hours a day, for 3 weeks. Significant improvement in gross motor function was achieved by all the children.

Sessions usually are under the supervision of licensed certified physical therapists, who had hands-on training in intensive suit therapy. The typical day routine consists of tissue massage and warm-ups, sensory integration techniques, proper movement patterns and body alignment, development of motor skills, strengthening exercises, and flexibility, balance, and coordination exercises, but each program may be different according to the therapist. Different rehabilitation techniques can be facilitated by using cables, pulleys, and weights. Children often exercise in safe exercise units, known as "monkey cages" or "spider cages," in which the pulleys and weights help to isolate movements, thereby strengthening the muscles.

Children with certain medical conditions, such as high blood pressure, heart and circulatory conditions, diabetes, kidney problems, severe scoliosis, hydrocephalus (VP shunt), and uncontrolled seizures, must take their doctor and therapist approval before using the suit therapy.

The cost of intensive suit therapy is an important factor to be considered [58]. It is not covered by most insurance companies, and unfortunately, families have to pay out of pocket to pay it. Because the treatment is still considered experimental, it is not covered by some insurance companies.

2.19 Hyperbaric oxygen therapy

Hyperbaric oxygen therapy gained a lot of interest in the medical community. Despite it is not approved as a treatment option for CP, some private offices offer it to their patients. Hyperbaric oxygen therapy (HBOT) is a chamber that supplies the bloodstream with 100% oxygen, while the patient is inside a pressurized chamber. When the patient is inside the chamber, the air pressure will be increased three times higher than the normal air pressure, allowing the lungs to hold on more oxygen [59]. Oxygen is carried by the blood into the body tissues, the extra oxygen can fight infection, and at the same time, the body will stimulate and release stem cells and growth factors. Extra blood oxygen will restore and correct the tissue function and blood gas levels temporarily.

Currently, results are mixed regarding the benefits of HBOT therapy in CP children. There is a feeling that it will be the future of CP treatment. There is a consensus that HBOT works best in CP cases secondary to a brain injury caused by a lack of oxygen, rather than a genetic or developmental cause [60].

Not everyone agrees about the benefits of HBOT. In fact, some doctors believe that HBOT may do more harm than good to CP children. Published studies for clinical trials of HBOT by the National Institutes of Health (NIH) indicated that despite a minimal decrease in children mortality with traumatic brain injuries, it also increased the chances of a poor functional outcome [61]. There was no significant difference between CP children who received HBOT and a placebo group in published research in the modern drug discovery and NHI. Two clinical trials for CP children, 3–12 years of age. One group received hyperbaric oxygen at 1.75 ATA of 100% oxygen. The second group received slightly pressurized room air. They had daily sessions for 40 days. Both groups showed significant improvements in the following areas: attention, memory, gross motor function, speech, and functional skills. The treatment is not covered by most insurance companies, which does not cover the treatment because it is not considered current, valid treatment for CP.

2.20 The Anat Baniel method and NeuroMovement

The Anat Baniel Method and NeuroMovement is a movement type and brain-based therapy that triggers changes in the brain. Anat Baniel is a psychologist and dancer who became interested in the relationship between movement, the brain, and wellness. She was Dr. Moshe Feldenkrais's co-worker and father of the Feldenkrais method. Her method is a type of movement therapy used to change connections in the brain and between the brain and body. She created a new unique approach to changing the brain based on this method and name it the Anat Baniel Method (ABM), also known as NeuroMovement. It uses movement to change the brain and stimulate its learning process and ability to adapt. Her team works with disabled children and adults after injuries and strokes. They work with healthy individuals such as athletes, musicians, and others to improve their performance.

Neuroplasticity, or brain plasticity, is the core of the treatment for the brain power to change in response to experiences [62]. The current belief is only infants can have neuroplasticity, which decreases significantly with age. Scientists for a long time thought that current research is proving this assumption wrong [62]. Good and bad changes could happen to the adult brains. Positive impact could happen at any age if this ability can be used, which is the bases of the ABM. The ABM identified certain conditions in which the brain can utilize its plasticity and create new connections and patterns. These are known as the nine essentials and underly NeuroMovement therapy [63].

1. **Movement with Attention.** Movement helps the brain change but only when accompanied by focus and attention on the body.

2. **Slow.** To learn a new activity, you must do it slowly. A slow pace focuses the brain and stimulates neural connections.

3. **Variation.** All learning requires variation. Therefore, children play as they develop. By trying all kinds of new things, they learn.

4. **Subtlety.** Movements and activities should be subtle so the brain can focus on minute differences.

5. **Enthusiasm.** By engaging in activities with enthusiasm and joy, the brain understands what is essential.

6. **Flexible Goals.** The way to achieving a target is not necessarily straight. As with children learning through play and experience, anyone using movement therapy tries many things and adapts as they go along.

7. **The Learning Switch.** The brain has either a learning or a non-learning mode. Effective therapy requires switching into learning mode.

8. **Imagination and Dreams.** To see changes, it is important to imagine and dream of the possibilities.

9. **Awareness.** You must be aware to learn. To trigger the brain to learn and change requires being fully present and aware of surroundings and the body's sensations.

Few research papers studied this method in CP children. There some studies and personal stories showed that ABM can reverse some disabilities. Different random movements can help a healthy baby to learn and develop. On the other hand, a CP child's movement is limited, which in turn limits development [63].

The trainer assists the child move in ways that will lead to positive brain changes and greater mobility [63]. The treatment goal is to fix certain body areas or physical defects. For example, spasticity and pain will be decreased by massage and PT for the legs, which in turn make the child's walks easier. ABM has a different approach based on the brain can learn and change, and the focus is on the brain not on one specific physical issue or defect at a time. As the primary organizing structure, the brain's ability to adapt impacts physical, emotional, cognitive, and social functions [63]. A child can overcome some of his/her disabilities caused by CP if the brain can change, learn, and form new neural connections. The therapy used by ABM practitioners replaces old neurological patterns with new ones [64]. An important aspect is that the ABM does not try to place children into predetermined developmental milestones. The approach treats each child's development as unique, and every child goes at his/her own pace.

2.21 Acupuncture

Acupuncture is an old medical practice that started in China almost 8000 years ago. In the United States, it is considered an alternative treatment and it must be studied more to prove its effectiveness, which might help CP children by reducing the child's symptoms and other associated disorders. The acupuncturists will insert tiny needles into specific areas of the skin. The Chinese mentioned, when the needle inserted in specific areas of the skin, it helps to release the body's life force, also known as the "qi" (pronounced "chee") [65]. Releasing the force will relieve pain, help treat illnesses, and improve disabilities. A University of Minnesota's team reported, the "qi" is located throughout the body with focuses in certain areas, including body fluids, actuation, body limbs, body's defense system, and eating, drinking, and breathing. Targeting pressure points, or meridians, within the body will trigger the qi. After inserting a needle into the pressure point, little pain will be felt by the patient, and he will feel qi moving throughout the meridians. When problem areas within the body were reached by the qi, it results in healing of the deficiencies.

Acupuncture therapy is relatively a new treatment for CP. Very few in-depth studies including NIH study have been done, but the results are encouraging. Acupuncture may provide great help to CP children and can help with the accompanying associated disorders. It can help with cognitive issues, hearing deficits, speech delays, imitations, pain relief, and improved gross motor functionality. The procedure is done at acupuncture clinics. Acupuncture is not one of the traditional treatment options to treat CP and we need more studies to confirm its effectiveness.

According to the National Center for Complementary and Alternative Medicine (NCCAM), "It is safe for children when therapy is performed by a well-experienced acupuncturist, but 2011 research concluded that a lot of side effects can occur when it is done by poorly trained acupuncturist" [66, 67].

The most side effects are dizziness, pain at the site entry, infections, nerve puncture injuries, fatigue, bruising, muscle twitching, and emotional release, which may lead to crying (this is generally a positive side effect). Bruising and nerve injuries are usually do not occur if the procedure done by a fully trained and licensed acupuncturist. To be qualified to practice acupuncture, the acupuncturist must attend a 3–4-year program accredited by the Accreditation Commission for Acupuncture or Oriental Medicine (ACAOM).

2.22 Medical marijuana

CP has a wide range of symptoms ranging from mild spasticity to the inability to control the limbs and uncontrollable. A lot of research has been done, but the focus is to find different treatments to help, control, or cure the symptoms. Research for studying medical marijuana in CP is limited. Previous studies suggest that it has some benefits, including pain control, reduction of spastic movements, reduction of seizures, and more.

A National Institutes of Health (NIH) study on pain treatment was published in 2011. The study enrolled 83 CP adults, treated with 23 different pain medications, including medical marijuana [68]. The most frequent painful areas reported were the legs, lower back, and hips. Results show that "Marijuana was the most effective treatment to relieve the pain; however, less than 5% of the patients never used it for pain relief."

The most severe form of CP is spastic quadriplegia, children cannot walk, and their speech is usually severely affected. While their extremities are spastic, the neck muscles may be weak, and they are not able to hold their head up. Pain and communication disorders are common in spastic quadriplegia. We have limited data and limited studies on the use of medical marijuana for spastic quadriplegia symptoms that showed multiple therapeutic benefits could be gained. An NIH published in 2007 on the clinical experience and animal studies demonstrates that the active constituents in marijuana help to control partial seizures, which are common in spastic quadriplegia [69]. A published study in 2014 studied the effect of marijuana in reducing painful muscle spasms in multiple sclerosis, which are very common symptoms in this patient group [70].

Cannabis oil or CBD oil, a derivative substance form of marijuana, has a lot of public attention in recent years, especially after a CNN program on a young girl who used to have more than 50 convulsive seizures per day. The family tried all available treatment options with no control over her seizures, and they used a formulation with a high concentration of CBD oil, now known as "Charlotte's Web" after their daughter's first name [71]. Her seizure's frequency went done to only 2–3 per day after they used the oil for weeks. Later, she was successfully weaned off her anti-seizure medications. She also started to walk, talk, and ride her bicycle, and she was not able to do all of them before. Now, CBD oil was sold by different companies as a treatment not only for CP children's seizures but also for muscle spasms and chronic pain. It is important to consult with your doctor and to search companies selling the oil before starting your child on any medications. Keep in mind, however, that some state laws and regulations do not allow your doctor to give you a recommendation for CBD treatment.

"Getting high" is a legitimate concern of families considering medical marijuana treatment for their children. According to the author of Stoned: A Doctor's Case For Medical Marijuana, THC is the compound in marijuana that makes people feel high [72]. THC is found in a very low concentration in most of the marijuana and cannabis oil used in medical compounds, and it does not get the patient high. On the one hand, euphoria and hallucinations are due to THC. You might get high if there is some THC in the marijuana you are using. On the other hand, CBD does not have any of those brain effects. There are some studies that used 300, 400, or 600 milligrams of CBD, which is a large dose with no bad psychological side effects. Medical marijuana and CBD oil generally contain a higher concentration of CBD, which help treat seizures and muscle spasms.

There are non-life-threatening symptoms associated with CP like speech repetition and stuttering. They prevent the patient to communicate more effectively. Speech disorders and impediments, such as stuttering in CP children, can be treated by medical marijuana. Despite the few clinical studies published on medical marijuana and stuttering, but many doctors advocate its use as an effective treatment option for speech problems. **L Assistance for Your.**

2.23 Stem cell therapy

Stem cell therapy is the new era of finding treatment for different disorders, including CP. Stem cells are body cells that can grow and change into other types of cells. Umbilical cord blood of newborns is the optimal option to access and use, and they can develop into nearly any type of cell in the body. Research gave us great optimism that stem cells can help treat brain disorders by regenerating damaged tissue. There are running clinical trials using cord blood to treat CP children. The results are very hopeful, showing that the use of the stem cells is safe and that it could be useful in treating CP symptoms. It may be proven to be a cure for the condition. CP is currently having no cure, but research is progressing, and emerging treatments are proving that there is hope.

3. Conclusion

To prevent cerebral palsy in infants and, thus, the resulting spasticity, it is important that mothers receive prenatal care during pregnancy, that measures are taken to avoid premature labor, and that special consideration is given to pregnancies involving multiple gestations. Early detection and treatment of neurodegenerative diseases may prevent the development of spasticity as well as detect the underlying diseases that could result in brain injury. If children have conditions that make them susceptible to brain or spinal cord injury or both, safety measures should be taken (i.e., helmets for patients who have frequent seizures). The goals of patient and benefits to the patient are important when considering the path of treatment. In some cases, function will not return, but treatment can result in pain reduction and allow easier management of patient care. Common goals are to decrease pain, prevent or decrease contractures, improve ambulation, facilitate activities of daily living, facilitate rehabilitation participation, save caregiver's time, improve the ease of care, and increase safety. Appropriate management choices are based on therapeutic objectives. Physical and occupational therapists can play a key role in identifying these objectives. Treatments with the fewest side effects are usually given priority. Both the patient's and the caregiver's goals must be considered.

4. Summary

A rehabilitation multidisciplinary team could be a good connection with management. Traditional treatments for spasticity include physical therapy, occupational therapy, and rehabilitation treatments, which complete a number of crucial tasks and specific goals in the treatment of patient with CP, this will promote their sensorimotor development, improve their overall posture and position, and enhance their control of movements in all their daily activities; a lot of physical therapy approaches were based on different theoretical principles though the main target is the management of abnormal muscle tone and improving the range of motion through neurodevelopment therapy, conductive education, constraint-induced movement therapy, etc.

Occupational therapy is a client-centered health profession concerned with promoting health and well-being through occupation, in which the patient is stretched anywhere from once daily to several times per day, but it has only a limited effect on the patient's spasticity. Rehabilitation treatment options include casting, orthotics or splints, strengthening, electrical stimulation, practice of functional tasks, sensory integration, muscle stretching, and targeted muscle training.

Oral medications can be used to decrease spasticity; however, many have unwanted side effects such as drowsiness, sedation, confusion, and fatigue. Benzodiazepines, such as diazepam, are rarely used because of their strong sedating effects. Other oral medications, such as anticholinergics, anti-seizures, address different issues related to CP children.

Speech therapy is recommended if the child has communication, swallowing, and breathing issues. It offers a wide variety of exercises aimed to help children communicate better, and it also addresses and helps in associated disorders that make speech more difficult.

Massage therapy has proven to offer mental, emotional, and physical benefits. It is a supportive therapy treatment in which the body's connective tissues and muscles are massaged and stimulated through direct contact by a massage therapist to promote healing and well-being in the patient.

Hippotherapy is another form of therapy that uses horses and equine equipment to help CP children to develop better physical functioning, as well as assistance with emotional and neurological functioning. Those therapies help strengthen muscles, improve balance and flexibility, and help your child with everyday living tasks.

Aqua therapy or aquatic therapy is a sequence of water-based exercises that help improve a person's physical abilities and functions. It is very useful for CP children because it allows the children to move freely without putting stress or much weight on their bodies. Several goals are to be achieved, including helping kids to develop more muscle control, increase self-confidence, improve strength and physical function, and gain more life independence.

Osteopathic manipulation therapy or OMT is a gentle manipulation of the musculoskeletal system that is supposed to relieve symptoms and improve overall wellness in patients practiced by a trained doctor in osteopathic medicine (DO). Studies results on how OMT can help CP children are mixed, and most of them are small or limited in some way, but there is some evidence that OMT can help CP children move better and feel better.

Chiropractic care for CP children is considered a natural type of treatment that can help with several musculoskeletal and nervous system conditions. Chiropractic intervention is done under a licensed chiropractor who will perform different techniques to help reduce pain and spasms and help to restore proper nervous system function.

Homeopathy is an example of modern alternative medicine such as traditional Chinese medicine, which has evolved over thousands of years. There are a lot of critics of homeopathy, but many people claim it has helped them get relief from symptoms. There are few, if any, risks of working with a trained homeopath.

Pet therapy, or animal-assisted therapy, is another way for CP children to get greater benefits from physical therapy sessions as well as other types of treatment. Working with animals is proven to be beneficial in many ways and, when added to standard therapies, can help children meet their goals. Pet therapy is the use of specially trained animals to promote wellness, boost mood, aid therapy, and other broad uses in mental and physical health care.

Pilates is a system of exercises using special apparatus, designed to improve physical strength, flexibility, posture, endurance, and mental awareness. It is easily adapted to all ability levels and can provide a strenuous strength workout for advanced athletes or a gentler workout for beginners, people recovering from injury, or those with physical disabilities.

Yoga is an ancient practice of mixing physical and spiritual elements. Many people around the world get benefits such as stress relief, flexibility, strength, and other health improvements. Yoga is also being used to help specific populations, like CP children and adults.

Functional electrical stimulation is developed originally to help people with paralysis, using electrical pulses to stimulate muscles, and it is now being used to treat a lot of medical conditions, including cerebral palsy. In CP children, it is proven to improve range of motion, muscle mass, muscle strength, walking speed, spasticity, gait, and foot and ankle positioning.

Chemo-denervation such as using botulinum toxin type A has proved easier, more effective, and less painful for patients. Botulinum toxin is a potent neurotoxin derived from the anaerobic bacteria *C. botulinum*, but when used in treatment, no serious systemic toxin effects have been reported.

Rhizotomy is used to decrease tone, increased mobility, and facilitation of care for the patient. However, the reduction in spasticity cannot be predicted and sometimes results in excessive hypotonia. Other neurosurgical approaches include peripheral neurectomy, myelotomy, and dorsal column electrical stimulation. Intrathecal baclofen pump therapy is a very effective treatment option for CP children.

Orthopedic procedures are the most frequently performed operations for spasticity. The targets of these operations are muscles, tendons, or bones. Muscles may be denervated and tendons and muscles may be released, lengthened, or transferred. The goals of surgery may include reducing spasticity, increasing range of motion, improving access to hygiene, improving the ability to tolerate braces, or reducing pain.

Intensive suit therapy is a new experimental therapy designed to help CP children by improving muscle tone, posture, and movement. Although more studies are needed to confirm its effectiveness in the long run. The intensive suit therapy consists of an orthotic suit that includes a hat, knee pads, and specially designed therapeutic shoes. It also has rings that allow bungee cord-like ropes to be inserted and adjusted according to the child's height.

Hyperbaric oxygen therapy is not recognized as a treatment option for cerebral palsy. Hyperbaric oxygen therapy (HBOT) is a chamber that provides pure oxygen into the bloodstream, while the patient lies in a pressurized chamber. While the patient is inside the chamber, the air pressure is increased three times higher than the normal air pressure, making it possible for the lungs to grab more oxygen.

The Anat Baniel Method and NeuroMovement is a type of movement and brain-based therapy that triggers changes in the brain. The ABM uses movement to change the brain and trigger its learning process and ability to adapt. Baniel and her team work with special needs children and adults with limitations, such as those caused by injuries and strokes. They also work with athletes, musicians, and others to help improve performance.

Acupuncture is one of the oldest medical practices. It is an alternative form of treatment in the United States and additional studies are needed to determine its overall effectiveness. Acupuncture may be used to lessen the child's symptoms and many associated disorders.

Medical Marijuana, cerebral palsy is a life-long disorder, with variety of symptoms ranging from mild spastic movements to the inability to control the limbs and severe seizures. Research on the use of medical marijuana in CP is still limited, but previous studies suggest that it offers a host of benefits, including pain control, reduction of spastic movements, reduction of seizures, and more.

Stem cell therapy is an emerging treatment for different conditions, including cerebral palsy. The umbilical cord blood of newborns is the optimal stem cell to be used. The results are very promising, showing that this emerging treatment is safe and that it may be effective in improving symptoms of cerebral palsy.

Author details

Yasser Awaad
Independent Scientist, Bloomfield Hills, USA

*Address all correspondence to: awaady@gmail.com

References

[1] Young J. Spasticity: A review. Neurology. 1994;**44**(suppl. 9):S12-S20

[2] Blair E, Cans C. The definition of cerebral palsy. In: Panteliadis C, editor. Cerebral Palsy. Cham: Springer; 2018

[3] American Occupational Therapy Association (AOTA). About Occupational Therapy. Retrieved from: https://www.aota.org/About-Occupational-Therapy.aspx

[4] Hoare BJ, Wallen MA, Thorley MN, Jackman ML, Carey LM, Imms C. Constraint-induced movement therapy in children with unilateral cerebral palsy. Cochrane Database System Review. 2019;**4**(4):CD004149

[5] Pandey K, Berman SA. What is the role of clonidine in the treatment of spasticity? Drugs & Diseases. 2019. Medscape Article

[6] Suárez-Lledó A, Padullés A, Lozano T. Management of Tizanidine withdrawal Syndrome: A Case Report (2018). 2018. DOI: 10.1177/1179547618758022

[7] Rabchevsky AG, Patel SP. Effects of gabapentin on muscle spasticity and both induced as well as spontaneous autonomic dysreflexia after complete spinal cord injury. Frontiers in Physiology. 2012

[8] Awaad Y, Rizk T. Spasticity in children. Journal of Taibah University Medical Sciences. 2012;**7**(2):53-60

[9] Hoda Z, Amy K. Cerebral Palsy Medication, Medscape, Drugs & Diseases, Neurology. 2018

[10] Vitiello B. Obsessive-compulsive traits in children and adolescents with Asperger syndrome. European Child Adolescent Psychiatry. 2010;**19**(1):17-24

[11] Cerebral Palsy Hope Through Research. National Institute of Neurological Disorders and Stroke | National Institute of Neurological Disorders and Stroke. 2020

[12] Santos-Longhurst A. Speech Therapy: What It Is, How It Works & Why You May Need Therapy. 2022

[13] Speech-Language Pathology and Audiology Certification. American Speech-Language-Hearing Association | ASHA. n.d. Retrieved from: https://www.asha.org/certification

[14] Alagesan J. Effect of modified suit therapy in spastic diplegic cerebral palsy – A Single Blinded Randomized Controlled Trial. Online Journal of Health and Allied Sciences. 2011;**9**:4

[15] Massage Therapy Can Help Improve Sleep. American Massage Therapy Association — American Massage Therapy Association | AMTA. n.d.

[16] Glew GM. Survey of the use of massage for children with cerebral palsy. International Journal of Therapy Massage Bodywork. 2010;**3**:10

[17] Pin TW, McCartney L, Lewis J, Waugh MC. Use of intrathecal baclofen therapy in ambulant children and adolescents with spasticity and dystonia of cerebral origin: A systematic review. Devotional Medicine. 2011;**53**(10):885-895

[18] Koca T, Ataseven H. What is hippotherapy? The indications and effectiveness of hippotherapy. PubMed Central (PMC). 2016. Retrieved from: https://www.ncbi.nlm.nih.gov/pmc/articles/PMC5175116

[19] Gorter JW. Aquatic exercise programs for children and adolescents

with cerebral palsy: What do we know and where do we go? International Journal of Pediatrician. 2011;**2011**:712165

[20] Wu DO, MPH P, J. A brief guide to osteopathic medicine. American Association of Colleges of Osteopathic Medicine. 2015

[21] Bertolino B, Kinder N, Cooper C. Effectiveness of osteopathy in the cranial field and Myofascial release versus acupuncture as complementary treatment for children with spastic cerebral palsy: A pilot study. Journal of Osteopathic Medicine. 2022;**122**(4):4149

[22] Tarsuslu T, Bol H, Şimşek İE, Toylan İE, Çam S. The effects of osteopathic treatment on constipation in children with cerebral palsy: A pilot study. Journal of Manipulative and Physiological Therapeutics. 2009;**32**(8):648-653

[23] Wyatt K, Edwards V, Franck L. Cranial osteopathy for children with cerebral palsy: A randomized controlled trial. Archives of Diseases Child. 2011;**96**(6):505-512

[24] Duncan B et al. Parental perceptions of the therapeutic effect from osteopathic manipulation or acupuncture in children with spastic cerebral palsy. Clinical Pediatrician (Phila). 2004 May;**43**(4):349-353

[25] American Chiropractic Association. About Chiropractic. What is Chiropractic? 2019. Retrieved from: https://handsdown better.org/about-chiropractic

[26] What is Chiropractic? Palmer College of Chiropractic. n.d. Retrieved from: http://www.palmer.edu/about-us/what-is-chiropractic

[27] Mayo Clinic. Chiropractic adjustment. 2018. Retrieved from: https://www.mayoclinic.org/tests-procedures/chiropractic-adjustment/about/pac-20393513

[28] Homeopathy. NCCIH. National Center for Complementary and Integrative Health. n.d. Retrieved from: https://www.nccih.nih.gov/health/homeopathy

[29] Seizure Disorders in Children. 2020. Retrieved from: https://thehomeopathiccollege.org/mr-muellers-articles/seizure-disorders-in-children

[30] Nimer J, Lundahl B, Therapy A-A. A meta-analysis. Journal of the International Society for Anthrozoology. 2015;**2015**:225-238

[31] Elmacı DT. Dog-assisted therapies and activities in rehabilitation of children with cerebral palsy and physical and mental disabilities. International Journal of Environmental Research and Public Health. 2015;**12**(5):5046-5060

[32] Said Kathie M. UCLA Health: High Quality Health Care Services, Top Health Care Specialists. Los Angeles, CA: UCLA; 2022

[33] Everything You Need to Know About Pilates. 2020. Cleveland Clinic. Retrieved from: https://health.clevelandclinic.org/everything-you-want-to-know-about-pilates/

[34] Egan MPH Little Movers: Pilates for Children with Neuromuscular Disorders. Balanced Body. Advance for Directors of Rehabilitation. 2006

[35] Veneri D, Gannotti M, Bertucco M. Using the international classification of functioning, disability, and health model to gain perspective of the benefits of yoga in stroke, multiple sclerosis, and children to inform practice for children with cerebral palsy: A meta-analysis. Journal of Alternative Complementary Medicine. 2018;**24**(5):439-457

[36] National Center for Complementary and Integrative Health. Yoga: What you need to know. 2019. Retrieved from: https://www.nccih.nih.gov/health/yoga-what-you-need-to-know

[37] Crow EM. Effectiveness of Iyengar yoga in treating spinal (back and neck) pain, International Journal of Yoga. 2015;**8**(1):3-14

[38] Singleton C. Functional electrical stimulation (FES) for children and young people with cerebral palsy. Paediatrics and Child Health. 2019;**29**(11):498-502

[39] Centers for Disease Control and Prevention. What is Cerebral Palsy? 2019

[40] Pool D. Daily functional electrical stimulation during everyday walking activities improves performance and satisfaction in children with unilateral spastic cerebral palsy: A randomized controlled trial. Archives of Physiotherapy. 2015;**5**:5

[41] Prosser LA, Curatalo LA, Alter KE, Damiano DL. Acceptability and potential effectiveness of a foot drop stimulator in children and adolescents with cerebral palsy. Developmental Medicine & Child Neurology. 2012;**54**(11):1044-1049

[42] Ahsanuddin S, Roy S. Adverse events associated with botox as reported in a food and drug administration database. Aesthetic Plastic Surgery. 2021;**45**(3):1201-1209

[43] Witmanowski H, Błochowiak K. The whole truth about botulinum toxin – a review. Postepy Dermatology and Alergology. 2020;**37**(6):853-861

[44] Shah S, Calderon M-D. Effectiveness of onabotulinumtoxinA (BOTOX) in pediatric patients experiencing migraines: A randomized, double-blinded, placebo-controlled crossover study in the pediatric pain population. Regional Anesthesia Pain and Medicine. 2021;**46**(1):41-48

[45] Mikov A, Dimitrijević L, Sekulić S, Demeši-Drljan Č, Mikov I, Švraka E, et al. Use of Botulinum toxin type a in children with Spastic Cerebral Palsy. Journal of Society for Development of Teaching and Business Processes. 2011

[46] Alvarenga A, Campos M. BOTOX-A injection of salivary glands for drooling. Journal of Pediatric Surgery. 2017;**52**(8):P1283-P1286

[47] Baricich A, Picelli A. Electrical stimulation of antagonist muscles after botulinum toxin type A for post-stroke spastic equinus foot. A randomized single-blind pilot study. Annals of Physical and Rehabilitation Medicine. 2019;**2019**:214-219

[48] Sargut TA, Haberl H. Motor and functional outcome of selective dorsal rhizotomy in children with spastic diplegia at 12 and 24 months of follow-up. Acta Neurochirurgica. 2021;**163**:2837-2844

[49] Summers J, Coker B. Selective dorsal rhizotomy in ambulant children with cerebral palsy: An observational cohort study. Health. 2019;**2019**:455-462

[50] Hägglund G, Hollung SJ. Treatment of spasticity in children and adolescents with cerebral palsy in Northern Europe: A CP-North registry study. BMC Neurology. 2021;**21**:276

[51] Stewart K, Hutana G. Intrathecal baclofen therapy in paediatrics: A study protocol for an Australian multicentre, 10-year prospective audit. BMJ Open. 2021;7(6)

[52] Skoog B, Hedman B. Intrathecal Baclofen dosage for long-term treatment of patients with spasticity due to traumatic spinal cord injuries or multiple

sclerosis. Annals of Rehabilitation Medicine. 2019;**43**(5):555-561

[53] Gottula A, Gorder K. Dexmedetomidine for acute management of intrathecal baclofen withdrawal. Toxicology. 2020;**58**(1):E5-E8

[54] Đapić T, Šmigovec I, Kovač-Đapić N, Polovina S. Surgery of cerebral palsy with special reference to treatment spastic luxation of the hip. Paediatrics Today. 2012;**8**:20

[55] Josenby AL, Westbom L. No support that early selective dorsal rhizotomy increase frequency of scoliosis and spinal pain – a longitudinal population-based register study from four to 25 years of age. BMC Musculoskeletal Disorders. 2020;**21**:782

[56] Pacific University Research. The effect of Intensive suit therapy compared to traditional physical therapy on gross motor function in children with cerebral palsy. 2010

[57] Bailes AF. Changes in two children with cerebral palsy after intensive suit therapy: A case report. Pediatric Physical Theraphy. 2010;**22**(1):76-85

[58] Karadağ-Saygı E. The clinical aspects and effectiveness of suit therapies for cerebral palsy: A systematic review. Turkish Journal of Physical and Medical Rehabilitation. 2019;**65**(1):93-110

[59] Mayo Clinic. Hyperbaric oxygen therapy. 2018. Retrieved from: https://www.amtamassage.org/approved position statements/Massage-Therapy-Can-Help-Improve-Sleep.html

[60] Wilson JL, Russman B. Hyperbaric oxygen therapy for cerebral palsy: Definition and principles. Cerebral Palsy. 2018;**2018**:1-9

[61] Goderez BI. Treatment of traumatic brain injury with hyperbaric oxygen therapy. psychiatric times. Psychiatric Times. 2019;**36**(5)

[62] Voss P, Thomas ME, Cisneros-Franco JM, de Villers-Sidani E. Dynamic brains and the changing rules of neuroplasticity: Implications for learning and recovery. Frontiers in Psychology. 2007

[63] Anat Baniel Method. Cerebral Palsy: How NeuroMovement Can Help. n.d. Retrieved from: https://www.anatbanielmethod.com/children/brain-trauma/cerebral-palsy

[64] Anat Baniel Method. Meet Anat Baniel. Retrieved from: https://www.anatbanielmethod.com/about/anat-baniel/meet-anat-baniel/

[65] Hafner C. What Is Qi? (And Other Concepts). n.d. Taking Charge of Your Health & Wellbeing. Retrieved from: https://www.takingcharge.csh.umn.edu/explore-healing-practices/traditional-chinese-medicine/what-qi-and-other-concepts

[66] National Center for Complementary and Integrative Health. 7 things to know about mind and body practices for children and teens. 2019

[67] Abbott R. Sensory rhizotomy for the treatment of childhood spasticity. Journal of Child Neurology. 1996;**11** (suppl. 1):S36-S42

[68] Hirsh AT. Survey results of pain treatments in adults with cerebral palsy. American Journal of Physics and Medical Rehabilitation. 2011;**90**(3):207-216

[69] Mortati K et al. Marijuana: An effective antiepileptic treatment in partial epilepsy? A case report and review of the literature. Review in Neurology Diseases. 2007;**4**(2):103-106

[70] Syed YY et al. Delta-9-tetrahydrocannabinol/cannabidiol (Sativex®): A review of its use in patients with moderate to severe spasticity due to multiple sclerosis. Drugs. 2014;**74**(5):563-578

[71] Young S. Marijuana stops child's severe seizures. CNN. 2013. Available from from: https://www.cnn.com/2013/08/07/health/charlotte-child-medical-marijuana/

[72] Bradley E. David Casinett's Stoned: A Doctor's Case for Medical Marijuana. Cerebrum 6-16. 2016

Chapter 3

Anatomical Surface Guided Techniques for Botulinum Toxin Injection in Spastic Cerebral Palsy Children

Raj Kumar and Shiv Lal Yadav

Abstract

Spasticity, a classical clinical manifestation of an upper motor neuron lesion, has been traditionally and physiologically defined as a velocity-dependent increase in muscle tone caused by the increased excitability of the muscle stretch reflex. Clinically, spasticity manifests as an increased resistance offered by muscles to passive stretching (lengthening) and is often associated with other commonly observed phenomena, such as clasp-knife phenomenon, increased tendon reflexes, clonus, and flexor and extensor spasms. If spasticity is not treated leads to abnormal posture, contracture, and painful deformities. This chapter will cover the botulinum toxin used in the management of spasticity while using the surface anatomy of upper and lower limb muscles. This will help enhance the use of this technique even in remotest setups where USG and EMG facilities are unavailable.

Keywords: spasticity, botulinum toxin, surface anatomy, cerebral palsy, upper limb, lower limb

1. Introduction

Cerebral Palsy (CP) is a combined disorder of movement, posture, and motor function often complicated or associated with various sensory, neurological, musculoskeletal complications, and behavioral problems. Nowadays, spastic CP is the most common type (more than 2/3rd cases) followed by dyskinetic, hypotonic, and ataxic. In spastic CP, diplegia is the most common (>50%), followed by quadriplegia, hemiplegia, and monoplegia [1]. Spasticity is commonly managed by stepped-up management protocol beginning with the more conservative options (exercises, physical modalities, occupation therapy, and orthoses) followed by oral medications (like baclofen, tizanidine, dantrolene, and tolperisone) and various surgical options for relatively older children at last resort, where stiffness and progressive deformities continue to hamper rehabilitative treatment. Chemodenervation by botulinum toxin-

A (BTx-A) decreases spasticity by denervating the muscle by inhibiting acetylcholine release from the neuromuscular junction [2]. It has a relatively focal, reversible effect with a wide safety margin. This BTx-A denervation temporarily reduces muscle tone and provides an opportunity to effect changes in motor learning and cortical motor organization [3].

BTx-A injection in the lower limb muscles may help in reducing spasticity, increase in range of motion, and improvement in gait pattern [4, 5]. BTx-A injection in the upper limb may also have favorable effects on decreasing the spasticity or resistance to passive movement of the spastic wrist and fingers and on self-care as an adjunct to other basic conservative means described above [6, 7].

In this chapter, we will be discussing surface anatomical or landmark-guided injection techniques in children with spastic cerebral palsy.

Most of the spastic upper and lower limb muscles can be injected by surface or anatomical landmark-guided technique. However, in the case of obese children or distorted anatomy, multiple times botulinum toxin injection ultrasound (US) guidance may be useful nowadays.

For surface anatomy or landmark-guided BTx-A injections, a common spastic pattern affecting the muscle and dynamic function is identified. In upper limb spasticity, the child has usually various combinations of isolated adducted and internally rotated shoulder, flexed elbow, forearm pronation, flexed wrist and finger, and thumb in palm posturing. Muscle injected commonly are pectoralis major, subscapularis, biceps, brachialis, brachioradialis, pronator teres & pronator quadratus, flexor carpi radialis & ulnaris, flexor pollicis longus, flexor digitorum superficialis, and profundus, adductor pollicis, opponents pollicis, and flexor pollicis Brevis. Whereas in the lower limb, any combination of hip in flexion, adduction, knee in flexion, ankle in equinus/equinovarus, flexed toes, and stiff knee on dynamic or static assessment.

For practical purposes, the injection site in the center of maximum muscle bulk usually lies in the midpoint of muscle or some cases between proximal one-third to the midpoint of muscle bulk. So, surface anatomical landmarks are midpoint or at maximum bulk and if another injection point is required, then a few centimeters proximal to this point depending upon the age and muscle involved.

1.1 Theory pearls

At muscle bulk there lies the end plate zone. Many past animal research has shown that injections close to these motor end plates are more efficacious [8] and in some muscles, it is also scattered throughout (sartorius, gracilis) [9]. As we cannot localize end plates by surface anatomy or clinical palpation. It is easy and practical to use surface/landmark-guided injection.

So, our target should be to identify surface landmarks, insert the needle in the belly (preferably midpoint and mid-thickness) of the muscle, and then gently stretch passively, needle movement is best appreciated if it is in the desired muscle. One should also ensure nil or minimal movement of the needle, while stretching other nearby/overlapping muscles or muscle slips.

In a few situations, we may have to use US guidance or US visualization for muscle identification and depth, then surface anatomical guidance may become more easier and precise. This is particularly required for deep muscles and relatively smaller muscles.

Otherwise, it might inject into undesired or neighboring muscles. As for any injection technique, we must ensure needle tips should not be in blood vessels or injure neural tissues.

Here, only commonly done lower limb and upper limb muscle is described in this chapter from proximal to distal joints/muscle and ease of doing the injection, which are as follows-.

2. Lower limb muscles

2.1 Iliopsoas

The child should lie supine on the edge of the table. Mark the inguinal ligament, palpate the femoral pulse, and now mark the femoral pulse line at the inguinal ligament. The midpoint of these two (obviously lateral to the femoral pulse) just below the inguinal ligament is the entry point of the needle. Passive extension of the hip on the edge of the table will show the movement of the needle, and adjust the depth accordingly. Prior US evaluation is better. For injection to be a more effective translumbar approach is required, authors do not advocate this injection without image guidance (**Figure 1**).

2.2 Adductor longus (AL)

The child should be in a supine position with hip and knee flexed. The spastic adductor will stand prominent in most cases in the anteromedial proximal thigh, while doing hip abduction. One can hold the muscle between the nondominant thumb and index finger and insert the needle at about proximal one-fifth to one-fourth of the muscle (**Figures 2a** and **b**).

2.3 Adductor magnus (AM)

If we want to inject (less practiced). The position will be the same as AL. At about proximal one-third of the medial thigh, just medial to gracilis. (Bony landmark 3–4 inch anteromedial to ischial tuberosity). The US is helpful because the needle may be in the gracilis or a medial hamstring if the needle enters a more anterior or posterior. Sometimes it may be deeper. Needle movement with passive abduction in knee extension/flexion confirms needle entry in gracilis or adductors (**Figure 3**).

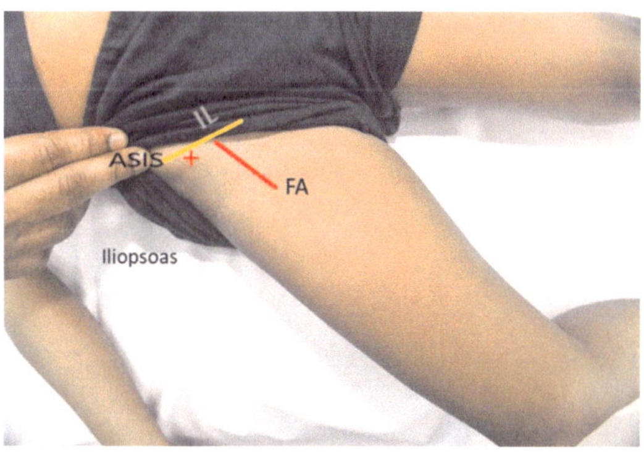

Figure 1.
Iliopsoas (IP): ASIS: Anterior superior iliac spine, IL- inguinal ligament, FA- line of femoral artery pulsation. Plus sign denotes the injection point.

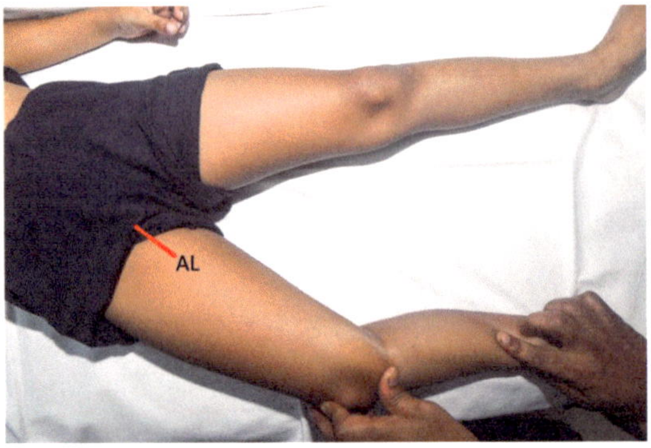

(a)

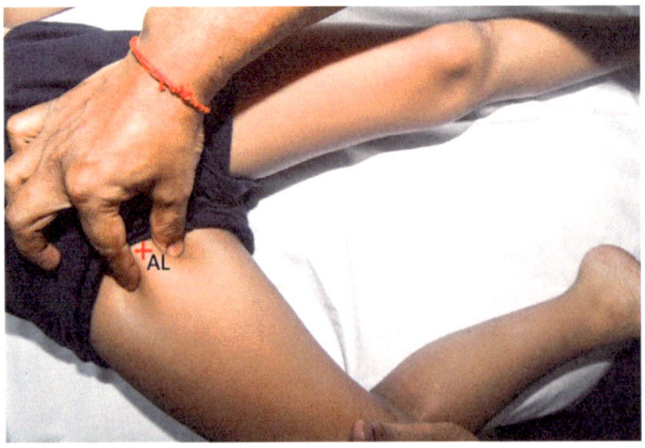

(b)

Figure 2.
a. Adductor longus(AL): red line denotes the prominence area of AL. b. Adductor longus(AL): plus denote vertical injection point, while holding the muscle in between fingers.

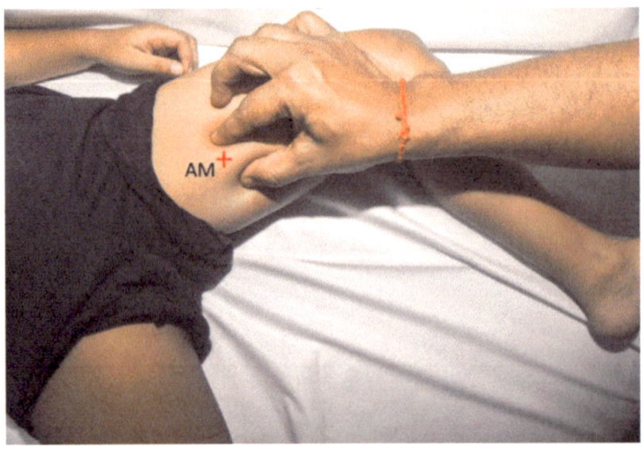

Figure 3.
Adductor Magnus (AM): in medial thigh inferomedial to AL point, at proximal one-third thigh plus demarcate injection point.

2.4 Semitendinosus (ST)

(Authors preferred approach) Patient lying prone with knee slightly flexed (already in most spastic patients) allowing terminal 30–40-degree extension or child lying supine with hip and knee 90-degree flexion. Now, the knee is extended as much as possible to mark and palpate the muscle. Now palpate the muscle at the junction of the proximal one-third distal and half of the thigh. It lies on the line joining from ischial tuberosity to medial post knee crease (tendon of semimembranosus) can be appreciated here. Here, we find the maximum bulk. Here, another point of injection 2–4 cm proximal to the previous injection point may be taken.

2.5 Semimembranous (SM)

Position and line same as semitendinosus. At the junction of proximal two-thirds and distal one-third, ST will be standing out prominently. Just medial to the prominent ST tendon. The injection is given. Passive extension of the hip in both positions helps in appreciating the good needle movement, thus confirming the muscle.

2.6 Biceps femoris (BF)

Same position as ST/SM. But the line changed. Draw a line between ischial tuberosity to lateral post knee crease (BF tendon is palpable). The midpoint of this line will be the target of needle entry. Palpate the muscle here by passive extension flexion of the knee. If one is confident, enter at the above-described midpoint for an injection. Caution should be taken for entry either medial or lateral to the tendon, the muscle may be deeper or even it may be congenitally absent. The needle movement must be appreciated. The US helps locate in case of difficulty (common with beginners) (**Figure 4**).

2.7 Rectus femoris (RF)

Make the child supine and draw a vertical line from the ant superior iliac spine to the center of the patella. The injection point is in the middle of it. It lies most superficial, just have to pass skin and subcutaneous tissue. So, adjust the depth accordingly. More deep needle insertion will go in vastus intermedius (**Figure 5**).

2.8 Gastrocnemius (GN)

The child should lie prone. Transverse mark the area/point where maximum calf bulk is there. Mark a vertical midline to differentiate the medial and lateral head. Now mark the lateral line corresponding fibular head and the medial line on the most anteromedial border of the tibia. The midpoint of the medial line and midline is the entry point of the medial gastrocnemius and the midpoint of the lateral line and the

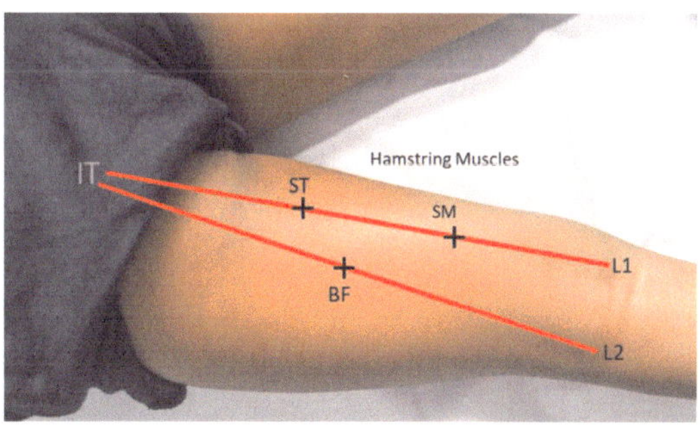

Figure 4.
Hamstring muscles: SM- semimembranosus, ST- semitendinosus, BF- biceps femoris. L1- line one joining ischial tuberosity to medial posterior knee crease. L2- line two joining ischial tuberosity to lateral posterior knee crease. Plus denotes the points of injection of mentioned muscle.

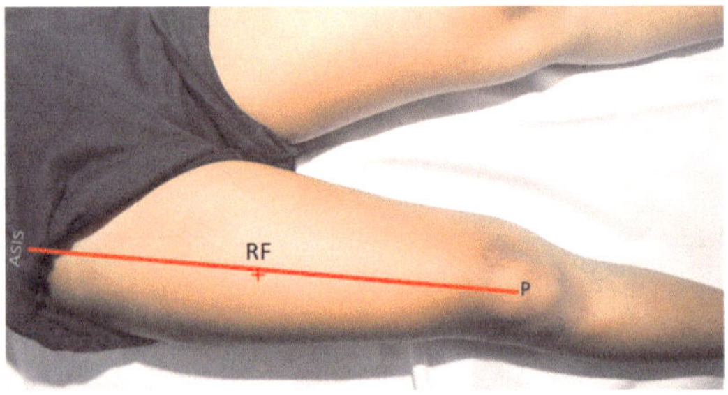

Figure 5.
Rectus femoris(RF): plus mark denotes injection point, which is middle of the line, joining ASIS and patella center.

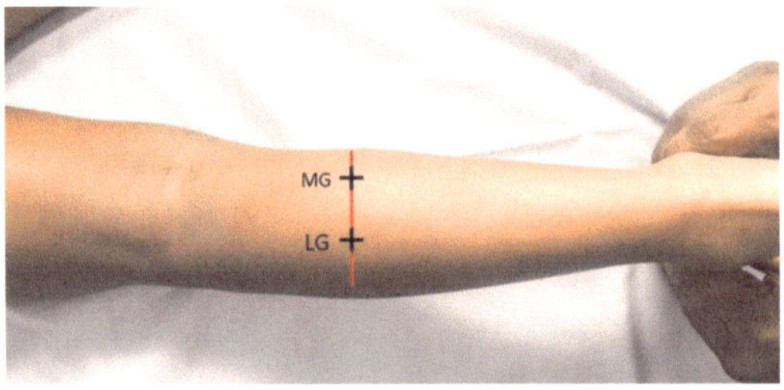

Figure 6.
Gastrocnemius(GN): line marked at the area of maximum calf bulk. Plus denotes the entry of the needle for MG (medial head gastrocnemius) & LG (lateral head gastrocnemius).

midline is the entry point of the lateral gastrocnemius. It is a very superficial muscle (needle vertical entry depth is only 0.5–0.8 cm in most children). Passive dorsiflexion beautifully elicits needle movement in both heads (**Figure 6**).

2.9 Soleus

The patient should lie prone, and look at the midpoint of the back of the leg. Between post knee crease and post upper margin of the calcaneus, where gastrocnemius lower margin is visible and palpable. One can inject just below the lower margin of the gastrocnemius. After needle insertion flexes the knee to 90 degrees (to avoid gastrocnemius action), and passively moves the ankle, good movement of the needle helps in correctly identifying the soleus. If the needle movement is less, may imply going deep into the flexor digitorum or tibialis posterior (**Figure 7**).

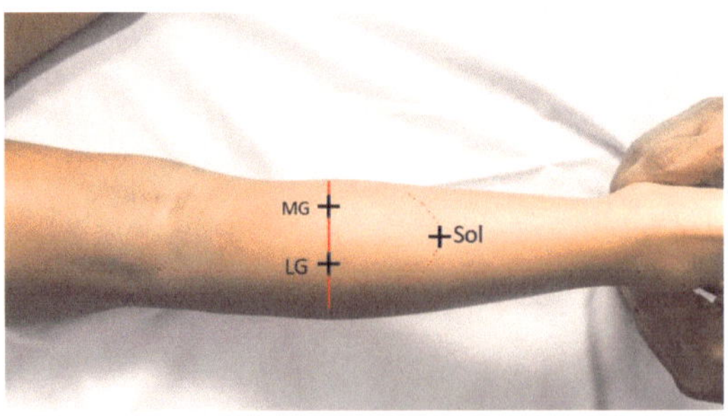

Figure 7.
Soleus(sol): plus denotes injection for sol at the lower margin of GN.

2.10 Tibialis posterior (TP)

Although we recommend US guidance for it, it may be injected with practice. The child should lie supine with hip and knee slightly flexed and externally rotated, so that the medial leg face upwards, Now just distal to the hallway of the leg, insert the needle just (0.5 to 1 cm) behind the tibia from the medial leg and advance it parallel to the tibia, first flexor digitorum Longus is traversed then will reach the tibialis posterior. Passive toe extension and flexion initially the passive eversion at the ankle will confirm the needle position.

2.11 Flexor digitorum Longus (FDL)

Positioning same as above (TP). In the mid-leg, this muscle lies anterior to soleus and posterior to tibia. Insert the needle at mid-leg just posterior to the tibia from the medial side and advance laterally parallel to the posterior tibia, It is the first muscle in the needle path, needle movement is appreciated well if we passively extend the 2nd to 4th toe. The needle will go in the tibialis posterior if we go more lateral. So, we can inject both FDL and TP in one go of a needle. If needle entry is more posterior, one can be mistakenly injected into the soleus (**Figure 8**).

2.12 Flexor hallucis longus (FHL)

The child should lie in a prone position, feet preferably hanging out from the bed. As we know this muscle crosses laterally to the medial from the upper two-third of the leg to the lower leg. At about proximal three-fourth and distal one-fourth junction of the leg just anterior to tendon Achilles tendon, one may insert the needle here and angle it toward laterally (aiming obliquely toward fibula), on passive extension of great toe, the needle should tilt/move. Adjust the depth accordingly. Prior US scans or guidance are helpful (**Figure 9**).

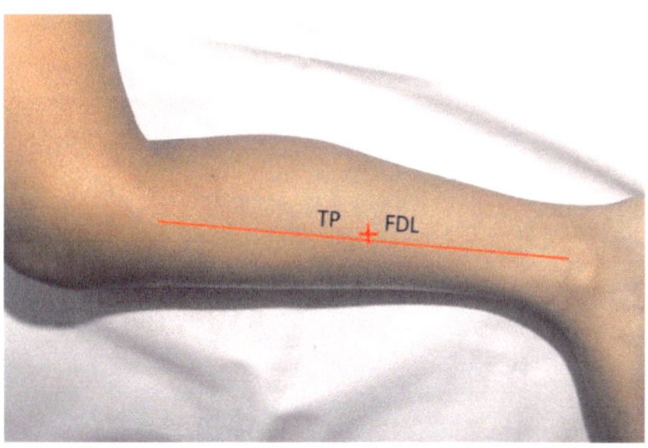

Figure 8.
Tibialis posterior (TP) & flexor digitorum longus (FDL): line is at the medial tibial border, plus is an entry point for TP& FDL injection (just posterior to the mid-tibia).

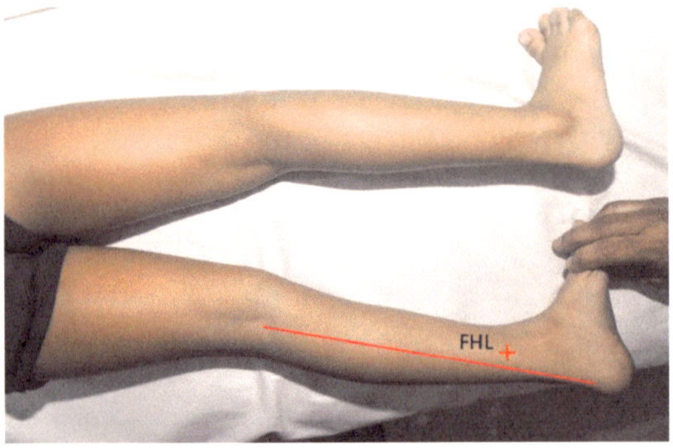

Figure 9.
Flexor hallucis longus (FHL): the line represents the length of the leg (post knee crease to tendo-achilles insertion), plus at the distal one-fourth anterior to tendon Achilles is injection point.

3. Upper limb muscles

3.1 Pectoralis major (PM)

Abduction of the arm to make it easily visible pectoralis. Hold it between your thumb and fingers. Then insert the needle, and try to give an injection from the single insertion in its upper, middle, and lower part by going tangentially. Take precaution to not go more medial and steep in very lean and thin children to avoid pneumothorax (**Figure 10**).

3.2 Subscapularis (SS)

Place the child supine. This muscle lies anterior to the scapula. So, mark the medial border of the scapula. At the proximal two-thirds and distal one-third junction of the medial border, the needle is inserted after slightly pushing the scapula posteriorly. The needle should advance laterally parallel to the scapular spine. Do not advance the needle anterior to avoid any pneumothorax. Once the needle reaches some distance, preferably near or less near to the center of the scapula. Somewhat needle movement may be appreciated if the arm is moved in external rotation (**Figure 11**).

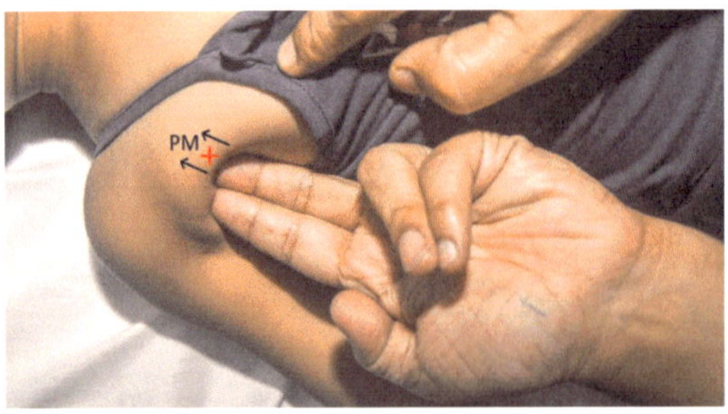

Figure 10.
Pectoralis major (PM): fingers elevating PM from anterior axilla, plus denotes entry point of a needle. Arrows depicting needle directions.

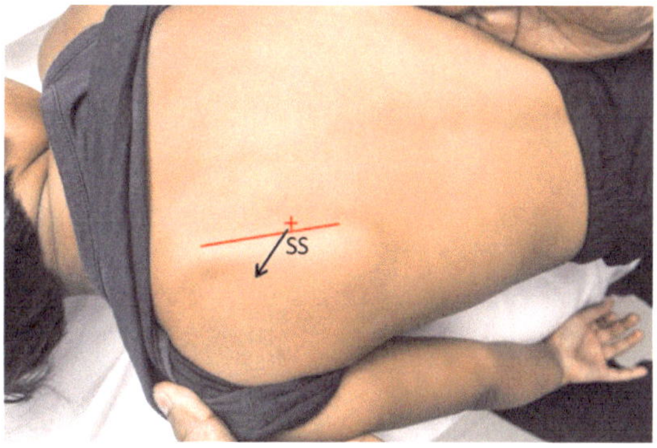

Figure 11.
Subscapularis (SS): plus at medial scapular border showing entry point for SS and arrow showing the direction of the needle.

3.3 Biceps

Child supine or sitting, arm by the side of the body, in elbow slightly flexed with the forearm in full supination. Palpate the anterior acromion point. Draw a line from the mid-elbow flexion crease (biceps tendon) and anterior acromion. The midpoint of this line corresponds to the center of the biceps belly. Muscle positioning may seem more medially in severe upper limb spasticity, such as adducted and internally rotated shoulder, so always take care of rotations and positioning. Hold the biceps between the nondominant thumb and index finger. Inject at this point. Passive slight extension and flexion will elicit good needle movement (**Figure 12**).

3.4 Brachialis (Br)

Positioning as for Biceps, mark the proximal two-thirds and distal one-third junction. At this point, find the place between the lateral border of the biceps and the lateral head of the triceps. Repeated supination and pronation will help in finding out the entry point, which is the first point/groove, where there is no biceps movement seen. Insert the needle at this point and push it further medically parallel to the transverse plane (toward the humerus). Pay attention not to go posterior to avoid entering in triceps. With the forearm in pronation passively gently extend flex the elbow a bit eliciting good needle movement (**Figures 13a** and **b**).

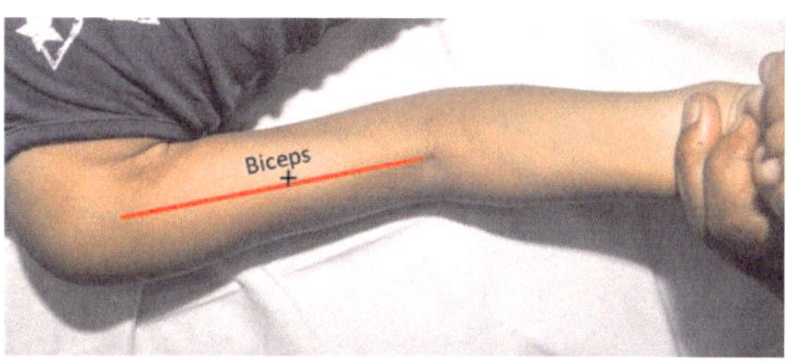

Figure 12.
Biceps: plus sign denotes the mid-muscle belly of the biceps as the injection point.

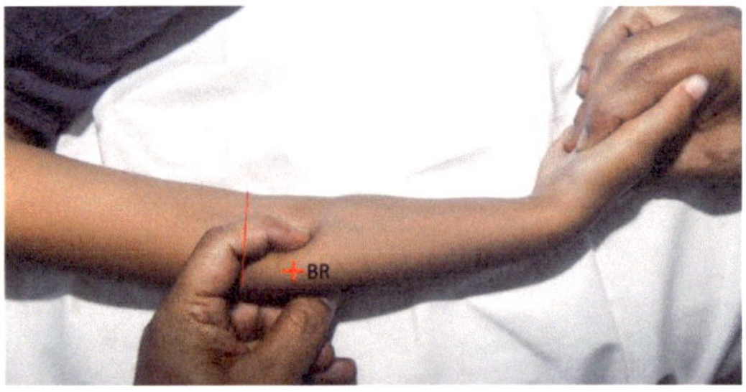

(a)

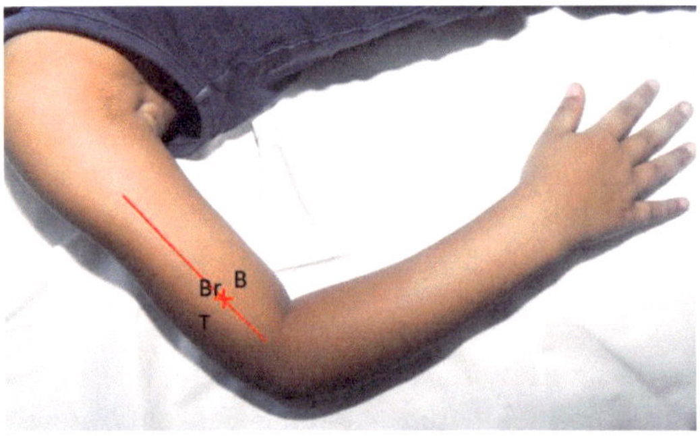

(b)

Figure 13.
a. Brachialis palpation: thumb in between lateral border of biceps and triceps. b. Brachialis (Br): B- biceps, T- lateral head of triceps, plus denotes injection entry point between B and T gap.

3.5 Brachioradialis (BR)

Supine position or cooperative child may be sitting with elbow 90 degrees flexed forearm in the mid-prone position. Now, keep the thumb in the antecubital fossa and index finger laterally to hold the muscle belly of brachioradialis between both fingers. At half to one inch distal to elbow crease, Insert the needle vertically down to reach a mid-depth of brachioradialis. Beware of posterior needle advancement, otherwise may inject extensor tendons. Passive elbow extension may show needle movement (**Figure 14**).

3.6 Pronator teres (PT)

The child should be supine or sitting as per convenience and cooperation with the forearm in supine. Take the midpoint of the elbow flexor crease and also mark the

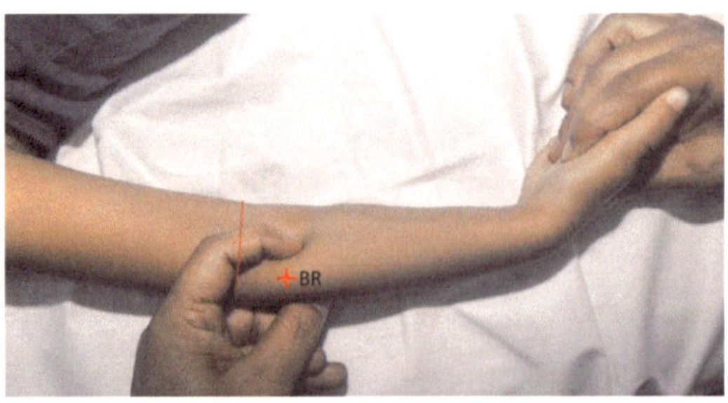

Figure 14.
Brachioradialis: line represents elbow flexor crease, forearm mid-prone, plus denotes injection for BR.

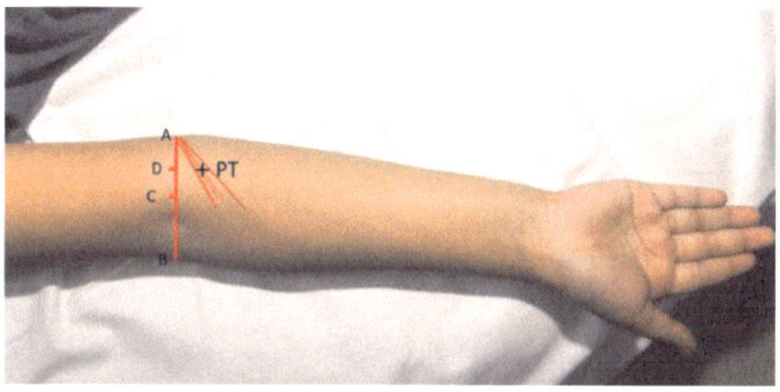

Figure 15.
Pronator teres (PT): A & B – medial & lateral elbow flexor crease, C – midpoint of A&B, D- the midpoint of A& C (junction of medial one-fourth and lateral three-fourth of elbow flexor crease).

lateral and medial points. Now, bisect the medial and mid-elbow crease points. Now, mark a point 1–2 cm distal to this point (medial one-fourth). Now place the index finger in the antecubital fossa, just medial to the index finger is pronator teres at the final mark point. Now, try to stabilize PT with the index finger and thumb, and confirm it by doing prono-supination. Now, insert the needle into it and again reconfirm the needle movement. If one is more medial and distal might inject into flexor carpi radialis, sometimes into flexor digitorum superficialis (**Figure 15**).

3.7 Flexor carpi radialis (FCR)

Positioning same as PT. Find out the apex of the cubital fossa. It is the point where the medial border of BR and lateral border of PT meet. Keep your index finger here. Palpate and try holding it between your thumb. Reconfirm it with the PT method by going 2–3 cm distal to the PT injection point. Good needle movement is appreciated by doing wrist radial-ulnar deviation and gentle passive extension (**Figure 16**).

3.8 Flexor digitorum superficialis (FDS)

Draw the first line between the mid-elbow flexor crease to the mid-wrist crease, second line from the medial epicondyle to the pisiform bone. Select the middle one-third between these two lines and make a rectangular box (as in **Figure 17**). Then, again divide this rectangle (with line 3) into equal medial and lateral halves. Now, 2nd finger FDS is more superficial at/near the distal part of 3rd line, 3rd FDS at the proximal part of 3rd line. 4th FDS and 5th FDS falls near just medial to 2nd line. 4th FDS superomedial to 3rd FDS and 5th FDS infero-medial to 2nd FDS. Avoid going near or crossing the first line laterally to avoid inadvertent injury to the neurovascular

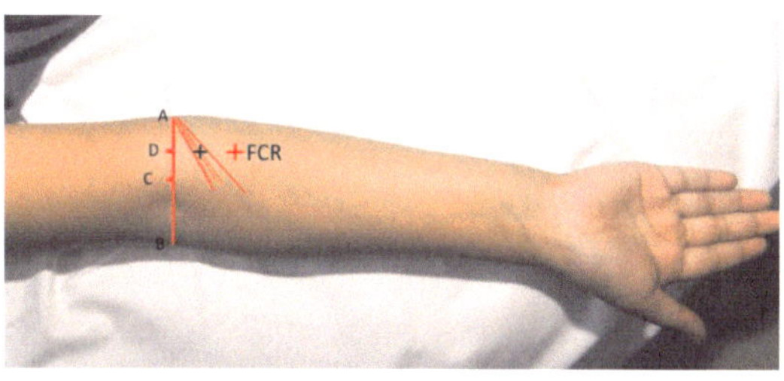

Figure 16.
*Flexor carpi radialis(FCR): A, B, C, D – as stated above in **Figure 15**. Distal plus sign denotes FCR injection point, proximal (left one) marked for PT.*

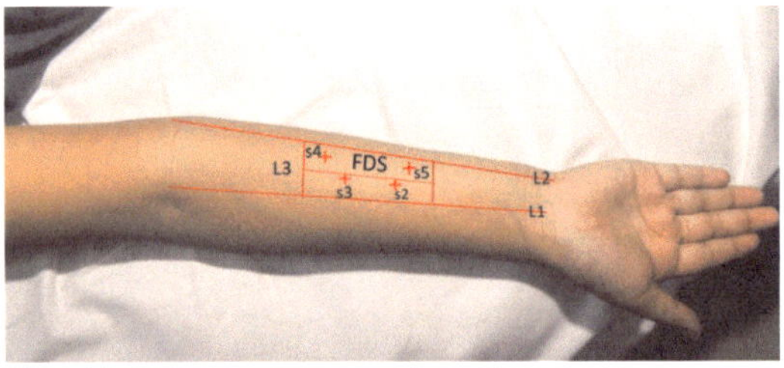

Figure 17.
Flexor digitorum superficialis(FDS): L1- the line between the mid-elbow flexor crease to the mid-wrist crease. L2- medial epicondyle to pisiform bone. The central big rectangle represents the middle one-third of the medial forearm. L3- equally divide this rectangle into equal medial and lateral half. s2- 2nd finger FDS, s3- 3rd FDS, s4- 4th FDS, s5- 5th FDS. Plus at s2, s3, s4, & s5 denoted vertical entry point for respective FDS slips.

bundle. So, we should focus on the medial rectangle. This is the author's practice method based on adult cadavers as described by Bickerton LE et al. [10].

3.9 Flexor digitorum profundus (FDP)

The child may be sitting on a chair with the elbow supported on the table or a child lying supine arm on the side of the body in some abduction. Elbow should be completely flexed, forearm in the mid-prone position. Make a line proximally from the olecranon to the distal medial wrist crease (line 1). The needle entry point is the needle entry point in the proximal one-third to the distal two-thirds junction of the forearm, just anterior to the ulnar shaft or midpoint between the ulnar shaft and line 1. Here, it traverses through flexor carpi ulnaris. So, we are more distal. We may inject it into FCU. So, inject between proximal one-fourth to proximal one-third. Passive extension of distal interphalangeal (DIP) joints will elicit the best needle movement. Individual fascicles may be injected with expertise and US guidance (**Figure 18**).

3.10 Flexor carpi ulnaris (FCU)

The child should lie supine or sitting with the dorsal forearm resting on the table in full supination. In the middle of the medial forearm, try to hold the muscle with fingers near/anterior to the ulnar border. Gentle wrist extension -flexion and radial-ulnar deviation should result in good needle movement. While finger

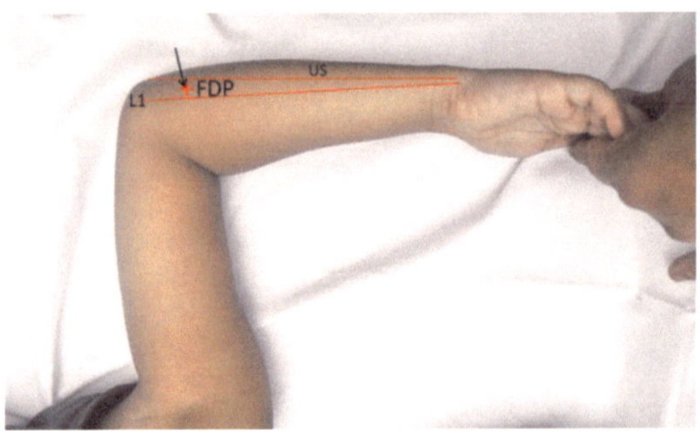

Figure 18.
Flexor digitorum Profundus (FDP): L1- line from olecranon medial wrist crease. US- line at ulnar shaft. Plus denotes needle entry point through the midpoint between the ulnar shaft and L 1 in proximal one-third to the distal two-thirds junction of the forearm.

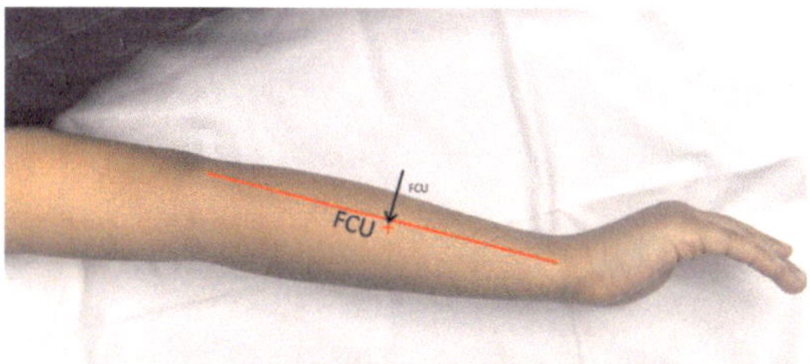

Figure 19.
Flexor carpi Ulnaris (FCU): line represents ulnar border. Plus denotes an injection entry point for FCU in the middle of the medial forearm. Arrow showing the direction of the needle.

flexion-extension should not show needle movement. Adjust the needle if one has gone anteriorly into FDS or deep into FDP (**Figure 19**).

3.11 Flexor pollicis longus (FPL)

Position supine or sitting. Forearm in full supination. Draw a line from the middle of the elbow flexor crease to the lateral wrist flexor crease. The middle point of this line is the area of interest. Also, start palpating the radial artery from distal to proximal. In the midpoint of this line, just lateral to radial artery pulse (almost lost at this point) is the needle entry point straight vertically downwards in mid-depth (skin to radius bone). Do not forget to aspirate, as the radial artery is very close. Passive extension-flexion of the thumb distally will help in the localization of FPL and movement of the needle confirms its placement in FPL (**Figure 20**).

3.12 Opponens pollicis

Supinated forearm means Palm facing up. Thumb adducted or thumb in the palm. Mark the midpoint of the thumb metacarpal. Gently aside the abductor pollicis brevis medially and insert the needle just medial to the bone from this midpoint and remain close to the bone. Gently move the thumb laterally (opposite action of opponens) to confirm needle movement and injection placement (**Figure 21**).

3.13 Adductor pollicis (AP)

Forearm pronated, palm facing down, thumb as much laterally as possible to make the dorsal first web as prominent as possible. Place one finger from the palm side and

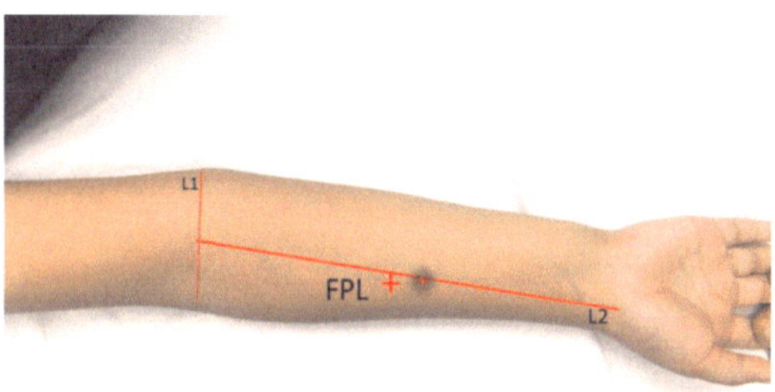

Figure 20.
Flexor pollicis longus (FPL): L1- line joining medial & lateral elbow flexor crease. L2 a line from MID PINT OF L1 to lat wrist flexor crease. Small plus (on line L2) denotes the absence of a palpable radial pulse. Larger plus lateral to it is a vertical needle entry point for FPL.

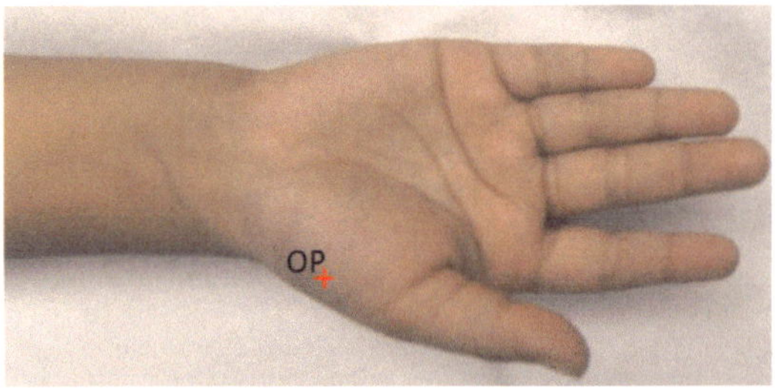

Figure 21.
Opponens pollicis: plus denotes the entry point for OP.

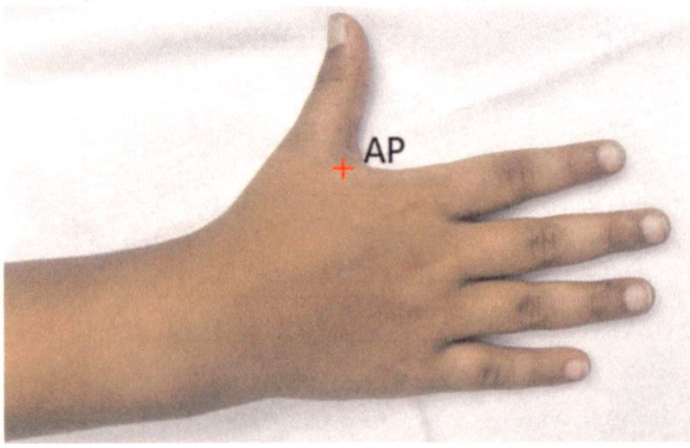

Figure 22.
Adductor pollicis (AP): plus denotes the injection point.

one from the dorsal side in between the first and second metacarpal to feel AP. Now, insert the needle in the center of palpated AP from the dorsal 1st web space (center), and adjust the needle depth accordingly (**Figure 22**).

3.14 Lumbricals

These are small muscles, that may be injected with sound anatomical knowledge, surface landmarks, or the US-guided. For the first lumbrical, the point marks the distal one-third and proximal two-thirds junction of the second metacarpal (radial side). At this, it lies just radial to this point. First, palpate the muscle by doing metacarpal flexion with distal joints in extension. Once palpated, inject at this point. Similarly, all others can be injected (**Figure 23**).

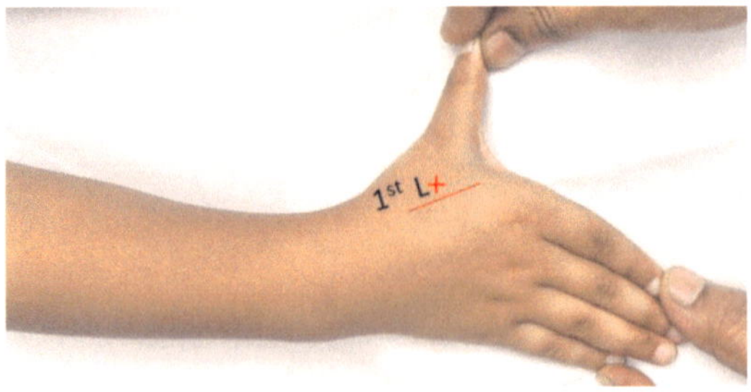

Figure 23.
Lumbricals: plus denotes the entry point for the first lumbrical (1st lumbrical), line represents the radial border of the 1st index metacarpal.

Author details

Raj Kumar[1]* and Shiv Lal Yadav[2]

1 Department of Physical Medicine and Rehabilitation, Indira Gandhi Institute of Medical Sciences, Patna, India

2 Department of Physical Medicine and Rehabilitation, All India Institute of Medical Sciences, New Delhi, India

*Address all correspondence to: drkrraj@gmail.com

References

[1] Kumar R, Gupta AK, Runu R, Pandey SK, Kumar M. Clinical profile of cerebral palsy: A study from multidisciplinary clinic at tertiary care Centre. International Journal of Contemporary Pediatrician. 2018;**5**: 1626-1630

[2] Koman LA, Mooney JF 3rd, Smith B, Goodman A, Mulvaney T. Management of cerebral palsy with Botulinum-A toxin: Preliminary investigation. Journal of Pediatric Orthopedics. 1993;**13**: 489-495

[3] Jefferson RJ. Botulinum toxin in the management of cerebral palsy. Developmental Medicine and Child Neurology. 2004;**46**:491-499

[4] Raj K, Sanjay W, Singh U, Yadav SL. A study of effects of intervention of Botulinum toxin- A on lower limb in children with spastic cerebral palsy. IJOPMR. 2015;**26**(4):94-101

[5] Kumar R, Wadhwa S, Singh U, Yadav SL. Clinical outcome with Botulinum toxin-A in spastic cerebral palsy children with equinus gait. Astrocyte. 2015;**2**:4-7

[6] Andringa A, van de Port I, van Wegen E, Ket J, Meskers C, Kwakkel G. Effectiveness of botulinum toxin treatment for upper limb spasticity poststroke over different ICF domains: A systematic review and Meta-analysis. Archives of Physical Medicine and Rehabilitation. 2019;**100**(9):1703-1725

[7] Farag SM, Mohammed MO, El-Sobky TA, ElKadery NA, ElZohiery AK. Botulinum toxin a injection in treatment of upper limb spasticity in children with cerebral palsy: A systematic review of randomized controlled trials. JBJS Review. 2020;**8**(3)

[8] Childers MK, Cornegay JN, Aloki R, et al. Evaluating motor end plate targeted injection of Botulinum toxin A in a canine model. Muscle & Nerve. 1998;**21**:653-655

[9] Aquilonius SM, Askmark H, Gillberg PG, et al. Topographical localization of motor endplates in cryosections of whole human muscle. Muscle & Nerve. 1984;**7**:287-293

[10] Bickerton LE, Agur AM, Ashby P. Flexor digitorum superficialis: Locations of individual muscle bellies for botulinum toxin injections. Muscle & Nerve. 1997;**20**(8):1041-1043

Chapter 4

Neurosurgical Treatment of Cerebral Palsy

Pinar Kuru Bektaşoğlu

Abstract

There is a broad range of alternatives in terms of cerebral palsy treatment (intrathecal baclofen (ITB), selective dorsal rhizotomy (SDR), and deep brain stimulation (DBS)). In order to reduce dystonia and spasticity, ITB bump insertion, SDR, and DBS are the main neurosurgical treatment approaches. In ITB treatment, a baclofen pump is implanted in the abdomen and is connected to spine via a thin tube. The pump is refilled regularly. It may require a replacement surgery. SDR includes cut of sensory nerves in affected site. Globus pallidus is the target in DBS surgery, the main advantage of this technique is that, it is reversible and adjustable. In this chapter, neurosurgical treatment alternatives for cerebral palsy will be discussed.

Keywords: cerebral palsy, deep brain stimulation, dystonia, intrathecal baclofen pump, selective dorsal rhizotomy, spasticity

1. Introduction

The International Executive Committee for Cerebral Palsy (CP) proposed the following definition: "*Cerebral palsy describes a group of permanent disorders of the development of movement and posture, causing activity limitation, that are attributed to non-progressive disturbances that occurred in the developing fetal or infant brain. The motor disorders of CP are often accompanied by disturbances of sensation, perception, cognition, communication and behavior, by epilepsy, and by secondary musculoskeletal problems*" [1]. This definition is supplemented by an interpretation of the terms used in the definition. CP can be defined according to the anatomical location of the brain lesion (cerebral cortex, pyramidal tract, extrapyramidal system, or cerebellum); clinical signs and symptoms (spasticity, dyskinesia [dystonic and choreo-athetotic forms], or ataxia); topographical involvement of extremities (diplegia, hemiplegia, or quadriplegia); timing of presumed insult (prepartum, intrapartum, or postneonatal); and classification of degree of muscle tone (isotonic, hypotonic, or hypertonic) [2]. Hypertonia, which is characterized by abnormal resistance to joint movement, is common in CP [2]. Spasticity, dystonia, rigidity or mixed subtypes are particular forms of hypertonia. Spasticity is the most common form of hypertonia, which is characterized by increased resistance to motion above a threshold joint speed [2]. The efferent output of alpha motor neurons regulates the muscle tone [3]. Dystonia is involuntary muscle activation causing abnormal posturing. Rigidity is resistance to motion independent from velocity, caused by simultaneous contraction of agonists and antagonist muscles. Treatment of CP targets the particular pathophysiology. In general, spasticity can be easier to manage than dystonia [4]. Studies on the management of spasticity are more abundant than those related to the management of dystonia in patients with CP.

There is an inverse relationship between the level of spasticity and voluntary motor control. In children with poor selective motor control, the spasticity can have functional importance (i.e. for standing). Treating this functional muscle tone may debilitate the child in everyday life [4]. Spasticity impairs selective motor control and treating it increases functionality.

The non-surgical treatment of CP includes enteral or intramuscular pharmacological agents, botulinum toxin injections, and physiotherapy [5]. When maximum tolerated dosage has been tried, neurosurgical alternatives such as intrathecal baclofen (ITB) therapy, selective dorsal rhizotomy (SDR), and deep brain stimulation (DBS) can be performed for the management of spasticity, muscle tone, and pain. The aim of neurosurgical interventions includes improvement in gross motor function, walking, muscle tone, health related quality of life, reduction of pain, and reducing the use of concurrent medication. In this chapter, we will review these procedures and provide up-to-date findings regarding neurosurgical alternatives in the management of hypertonia in CP.

2. Intrathecal baclofen pump

Intrathecal baclofen pump placement is a cost-effective treatment modality in spasticity and dystonia management of patients with CP that are non-responsive to enteral pharmacological treatments [6]. Penn and Kroin were the first scientists using ITB to treat spasticity in patients with multiple sclerosis [7]. Baclofen is a chlorophenol derivative of the inhibitory neurotransmitter gamma-aminobutyric acid (GABA) [3]. Intrathecal administration of this product results in ten times the concentration after oral administration [3]. Direct administration of baclofen to central nervous system via intrathecal route minimizes dosage and decreases systemic side effects when compared with oral form of baclofen [6]. ITB disseminates into the superficial layers of the spinal cord and binds to $GABA_b$ receptor sites, and acts presynaptically. It inhibits the uptake of calcium and inhibits the release of excitatory neurotransmitters (i.e. glutamic acid and aspartic acid) [3]. A single dose of ITB reduces lower extremity muscle tone within 20–40 min, its maximum effect is seen in 4 h after administration. Its half-life is 5 h and a single dose is effective for 8–10 h. ITB treatment improves muscle tone, gait, and quality of life of patient with CP. Approximately 300 μg/day dose of ITB is mostly adequate in reducing lower extremity spasticity and diminishing muscle spasms [3]. ITB overdose results in coma, respiratory depression, and hypotonia [3]. These effects usually subside within 2–3 days. Intravenous physostigmine is the treatment of choice in ITB overdose, however severe overdoses are not reversed.

Continuous ITB is best achieved via a pump which delivers baclofen to the lumbar area of the spinal cord to reduce spasticity in the lower extremities [8]. The catheter is inserted through means of a 14-gauge Tuohy needle and enters the spinal canal at about L2, and the tip of the catheter is advanced to T10 for paraplegics, T5 for quadriplegics, and C5-T1 for complex movement disorders and dystonia [9]. Right lower quadrant of the abdomen is the usual side for subcutaneous pump placement. A catheter is passed from the pump into the intrathecal space. Baclofen dose can be arranged via a radiofrequency wand which transmits information from a computer to the implanted pump [10]. Test dose is needed in the preimplantation period before the procedure. This will help physician to assess the potential effects of baclofen on symptoms and function. The initial continuous infusion dose is mostly twice the single ITB dose that shows a clinically prominent effect. The daily dose is slowly increased until desired clinical effects are present. Regular follow-up and percutaneous pump refill every three to six months is a requirement for this procedure. The pump is refilled by inserting a needle through the skin into the reservoir. Frequent monitoring and dose adjustment is a must after pump placement. Pump replacement is also a necessity at the end of battery life (4–6.5 years). The pump is similar to hockey pump, and the child must weigh approximately 15–18 kg to accommodate the pump. ITB affects both spasticity and dystonia and benefits both ambulatory and non-ambulatory children.

Shared decision-making between physician and patient and his/her caregivers is an important step. The adverse events include CSF leakage, infection, catheter disconnection or breakage, constipation, respiratory depression, baclofen withdrawal, and baclofen overdose [5, 10]. Highest complications rates for ITB therapy are around 36% [11]. Baclofen withdrawal symptoms include muscle spasms, dysesthesias, pruritus, agitation, and rhabdomyolysis. Treatment of this issue is restoring the ITB delivery [6]. Contraindications are baclofen sensitivity, inappropriate body size for reservoir placement, non-compliant patient, or any limitation that inhibits close follow-up. In patients with unilateral spasticity, ITB would probably also decrease muscle tone on the healthy side and ITB is not recommended for these patient group. Benefits and risks associated with ITB treatment should be cautiously evaluated; individual needs, expectations, and clear treatment goals should be agreed before procedure. Children with moderate to severe spasticity spectrum will benefit from ITB.

3. Rhizotomies

3.1 Selective dorsal rhizotomy

Normal cerebral inhibitions of the monosynaptic reflex arc at the spinal cord level are lost in children with spasticity from CP. This results with spasticity or hyperreflexia. Spasticity can be diminished via disrupting this hyperactive monosynaptic reflex arc [8]. At the dorsal root level, selectively transecting the afferent sensory fibers can significantly decrease spasticity. After lumbar laminectomy, the dorsal rootlets are localized in the cauda equina. Lumbosacral spinal sensory nerve rootlets with abnormal thresholds to electromyographic stimulation are sectioned to solve the sensory dysfunction in spasticity [6]. These are the afferent dorsal rootlets that terminate on relatively uninhibited alpha motor neurons [3]. When sectioned, spasticity can be relieved without losing other functions of dorsal roots. An abnormal response is considered when a muscle, not typically innervated at that root level, responds or when several muscle groups respond simultaneously [8]. Usually, 50% of the rootlets are cut [12]. The percentage of rootlets cut does not necessarily correspond to the level of spasticity or severity of neurologic involvement. Following the rhizotomy, there is a temporary weakness which returns to normal in few months. The other risks for this procedure are loss of bladder and bowel control, sensory loss, wound infection and meningitis, and finally leakage of the spinal fluid through the wound. Best candidates for SDR are children with spastic diplegia, ambulatory, pure spastic, cognitively intact, and with good social structure [8]. SDR only resolves spasticity with no effect on dystonia. Children with quadriplegic CP may not benefit from SDR because of their significant dystonia. Contraindications are spasticity of spinal cord origin, athetosis, rigidity, history of previous tendon release/lengthening, poor trunk control, severe weakness.

Selective dorsal (posterior) rhizotomy is a costly, irreversible complex neurosurgical procedure to reduce muscle tone in patients with CP. There is concern for muscle weakness, spinal deformity, and need for additional orthopedic procedures. Evaluation of multidisciplinary team when deciding to perform SDR is a must. Birth history, neuroimaging, strength, selective motor control, gait analysis, and presence of fixed deformities should be considered beforehand [13]. This procedure should be reserved for the patient population who does not respond or tolerate the pharmacological treatments and meet specific selection criteria. Also this procedure should be performed by a specialist multidisciplinary team with expertise in the management of spasticity. Intensive physiotherapy is mostly required for several months after procedure because the sensory input is reduced to sensory-motor reflex arcs in the spinal cord. Walking ability may be disrupted and different walking skills may be needed after the procedure.

Long-term follow-up studies report that SDR is well-tolerated over the years and improves functional outcomes and quality of life [13–15]. Daunter et al. reported less decline in gross motor function and required less hours of assistance in daily activities, however there was no difference for pain and fatigue [16]. Munger et al. reported improved gait quality in ten-year follow-up study [17]. In that study, non-SDR group required more orthopedic interventions and injections. Quality of life or functional and mobility measures did not differ among SDR and non-SDR groups.

3.2 Ventral rhizotomy

In the presence of mixed tone, ventral rhizotomy (VR) may be performed in conjunction with SDR when there is limited access to ITB and DBS [6]. SDR inhibits the sensory dysfunction leading to spasticity, while VR aims to solve the motor abnormalities associated with dystonia. Using this procedure in diplegic/quadriplegic children with CP with mixed spasticity and dystonia, [18] reported improved joint range of motion, spasticity, and dystonia at one-year follow-up. Functional intraoperative monitoring is crucial for identifying the roots to preserve sphincter innervation. This combined intervention may have promise in children with severe mixed hypertonia.

4. Deep brain stimulation

Deep brain stimulation may also be indicated in patient that are not responsive to ITB therapy [19]. Electrodes are placed in the basal ganglia and connected to an implanted pulse generator. Basal ganglia and thalamocortical network modulation are targeted. The stimulation can be unilateral or bilateral [9]. In a study targeting internal globus pallidus, there was 33% reduction in dystonia measures at one-year follow-up [20]. Parkinson disease and congenital dystonia are 2 movement disorders with very good outcomes from DBS. Acquired dystonias, from CP and after brain injury, are very heterogeneous lesions, isolated excellent results have been obtained with DBS in those cases, but criteria for patient selection remain uncertain [9]. DBS is reserved for patients with significant functional limitations who failed all other interventions for severe generalized dystonia [21–23].

5. Discussion

Cerebral palsy is characterized by motor dysfunction due to lesion occurring non-progressive disorders of posture and movement caused by injury to the infant or developing fetal brain [1]. Neuromuscular and musculoskeletal problems such as spasticity, dystonia, muscle contractures, abnormal bone growth, poor balance, weakness, and loss of selective motor control are some of the main problems encountered by the patients with CP. Physical and occupational therapy, bracing, oral medications, neurolytic blocks, neurosurgical procedures, orthopedic surgery, and others are the treatment alternatives [4]. These modalities do not cure the disease but improve function and improve quality of life. A multidisciplinary team should evaluate the patient and optimize the treatment. Neurosurgeons also play an important role in this team. Focal spasticity can be treated via lesioning the nerve target [24]. ITB therapy is the first choice in patient that are not responsive to enteral and physical treatments. Ambulatory children with spastic diplegia and good cognitive abilities can be treated with SDR. In a non-functioning limb, dorsal root entry zone lesioning could be an option for severe cases. DBS can be effective in the treatment of primary dystonias (especially those caused by DYT-1 gene mutation [25].

The evidence for recommending neurosurgical procedures (ITB pumps and SDR) is limited and of low quality [5, 26]. Recommendation of these procedures depend on the experience and expertise of the multidisciplinary team. It should be a shared decision-making between surgeon, patient and caregiver. Reported adverse events for ITB pump are catheter or pump infections, battery failure, catheter leakage, baclofen withdrawal or overdose, constipation, anxiety or depression, and seizures. These modalities are considered as complex and invasive. There is a need for high quality evidence for the neurosurgical treatment of CP. Clear expectations and open treatment aims should be discussed before the final decision step.

6. Conclusion

Neurosurgical procedures (ITB, SDR, and DBS) are invasive and costly procedures for the treatment of hypertonia in patients with CP. These modalities are not preferred in the first stage of treatment selection. However, they are considered a second step options for non-responsive patients with CP to other treatments modalities because they improve the major symptoms related to CP. These procedures are accepted as risky but in well-selected cases these modalities could have a real impact on patient's quality of life. High quality randomized controlled clinical trials are necessary to recommend these procedures for selected cases.

Conflict of interest

"The authors declare no conflict of interest."

Author details

Pinar Kuru Bektaşoğlu
Department of Neurosurgery, Sivas Numune Hospital, Sivas, Turkiye

*Address all correspondence to: drpinarkuru@gmail.com

References

[1] Rosenbaum P, Paneth N, Leviton A, et al. A report: The definition and classification of cerebral palsy April 2006. Developmental Medicine and Child Neurology. Supplement. 2007;**109**:8-14

[2] Sanger TD, Delgado MR, Gaebler-Spira D, et al. Task Force on Childhood Motor D. Classification and definition of disorders causing hypertonia in childhood. Pediatrics. 2003;**111**:e89-e97

[3] Albright AL. Neurosurgical treatment of spasticity: Selective posterior rhizotomy and intrathecal baclofen. Stereotactic and Functional Neurosurgery. 1992;**58**(1-4):3-13. DOI: 10.1159/000098964

[4] Gormley ME Jr. Treatment of neuromuscular and musculoskeletal problems in cerebral palsy. Pediatric Rehabilitation. 2001;**4**(1):5-16. DOI: 10.1080/13638490151068393

[5] National Guideline Alliance (UK). Management of Abnormal Muscle Tone: Neurosurgical Procedures to Reduce Spasticity: Cerebral Palsy in Adults: Evidence review A2. London: National Institute for Health and Care Excellence (NICE); 2019

[6] Nahm NJ, Graham HK, Gormley ME Jr, Georgiadis AG. Management of hypertonia in cerebral palsy. Current Opinion in Pediatrics. 2018;**30**(1):57-64. DOI: 10.1097/MOP.0000000000000567

[7] Penn RD, Kroin JS. Intrathecal baclofen alleviates spinal cord spasticity. Lancet. 1984;**i**:1078

[8] Young R. Drug therapy: Spasticity (first of two parts). New England Journal of Medicine. 1981;**304**:28-33

[9] Lynn AK, Turner M, Chambers HG. Surgical management of spasticity in persons with cerebral palsy. PM & R: The Journal of Injury, Function, and Rehabilitation. 2009;**1**(9):834-838. DOI: 10.1016/j.pmrj.2009.07.016

[10] Steinbok P. Selection of treatment modalities in children with spastic cerebral palsy. Neurosurgical Focus. 2006;**21**(2):e4. DOI: 10.3171/foc.2006.21.2.5

[11] Albright AL, Turner M, Pattisapu JV. Best-practice surgical techniques for intrathecal baclofen therapy. Journal of Neurosurgery. 2006;**104**(Suppl. 4): 233-239

[12] Agrawal M, Samala R, Doddamani R, Agrawal D, Chandra SP. The role of selective dorsal rhizotomy in the management of post-traumatic spasticity: Systematic review. Neurosurgical Review. 2021;**44**(1):213-221. DOI: 10.1007/s10143-020-01255-w

[13] Trost JP, Schwartz MH, Krach LE. et al, Comprehensive short-term outcome assessment of selective dorsal rhizotomy. Developmental Medicine and Child Neurology. 2008;**50**:765-771

[14] Langerak NG, Tam N, Vaughan CL, et al. Gait status 17-26 years after selective dorsal rhizotomy. Gait & Posture. 2012;**35**:244-249

[15] Park TS, Liu JL, Edwards C. et al, Functional outcomes of childhood selective dorsal rhizotomy 20 to 28 years later. Cureus. 2017;**9**:e1256

[16] Daunter AK, Kratz AL, Hurvitz EA. Long-term impact of childhood selective dorsal rhizotomy on pain, fatigue, and function: A case-control study.

Developmental Medicine and Child Neurology. 2017;**59**:1089-1095

[17] Munger ME, Aldahondo N, Krach LE, et al. Long-term outcomes after selective dorsal rhizotomy: A retrospective matched cohort study. Developmental Medicine and Child Neurology. 2017;**59**:1196-1203

[18] Abdel Ghany WA, Nada M, Mahran MA, et al. Combined anterior and posterior lumbar rhizotomy for treatment of mixed dystonia and spasticity in children with cerebral palsy. Neurosurgery. 2016;**79**:336-344

[19] Koy A, Timmermann L. Deep brain stimulation in cerebral palsy: Challenges and opportunities. European Journal of Paediatric Neurology. 2017;**21**:118-121

[20] Alterman RL, Tagliati M. Deep brain stimulation for torsion dystonia in children. Childs Nervous System. 2007;**23**:1033-1040

[21] Deon LL, Gaebler-Spira D. Assessment and treatment of movement disorders in children with cerebral palsy. The Orthopedic Clinics of North America. 2010;**41**(4):507-517. DOI: 10.1016/j.ocl.2010.06.001

[22] Fehlings D, Brown L, Harvey A, Himmelmann K, Lin JP, Macintosh A, et al. Pharmacological and neurosurgical interventions for managing dystonia in cerebral palsy: A systematic review. Developmental Medicine and Child Neurology. 2018;**60**(4):356-366. DOI: 10.1111/dmcn.13652

[23] Sanger TD. Deep brain stimulation for cerebral palsy: Where are we now? Developmental Medicine and Child Neurology. 2020;**62**(1):28-33. DOI: 10.1111/dmcn.14295

[24] Madsen PJ, Isaac Chen HC, Lang SS. Neurosurgical Approaches. Physical Medicine and Rehabilitation Clinics of North America. 2018;**29**(3):553-565. DOI: 10.1016/j.pmr.2018.04.002

[25] Volkmann J, Benecke R. Deep brain stimulation for dystonia: Patient selection and evaluation. Movement Disorders. 2002;**17**(Suppl 3):S112-S115. DOI: 10.1002/mds.10151

[26] Bohn E, Goren K, Switzer L, Falck-Ytter Y, Fehlings D. Pharmacological and neurosurgical interventions for individuals with cerebral palsy and dystonia: A systematic review update and meta-analysis. Developmental Medicine and Child Neurology. 2021 Sep;**63**(9):1038-1050. DOI: 10.1111/dmcn.14874

Section 3

Social Aspects of Cerebral Palsy

Chapter 5

Impact of Cerebral Palsy on Parents and Families

Marian Sankombo

Abstract

Cerebral palsy (CP) is a societal problem that may pose significant challenges and unique opportunities not only for the individuals with CP but also for their care givers, families, and siblings. It is the most common pediatric disability causing long-term functional limitations. The impact of CP on parents, families as well as sibling is evident in the level of stress, anxiety and depression envisaged especially on mothers. Siblings of individuals with cerebral palsy also suffers stigmatization that often result in social isolation. The presence of a child with cerebral palsy in any family can pose serious concerns to family relationships. Therefore, it is of utmost important to value the contribution of every family member, parents, siblings towards any planned intervention for a child with CP as they are affected by the disability in one way or another. This chapter explores the impact of CP on individual parent, families. Siblings as well as financial constraints associated with raising a child with CP.

Keywords: cerebral palsy, impact, parents, families

1. Introduction

The birth of a baby is a crucial event in the life of every human being. The dream of every parent becomes a nightmare if the baby they were expecting is born with cerebral palsy (CP). It is a complex neurodevelopmental disorder and is the leading cause of physical disability in childhood [1]. The condition affects body movement, muscle control, muscle coordination, muscle tone, reflex, posture and balance. A child with CP suffers from several conditions, ranging from spastic paralysis, cognitive, speech and visual impairment, chronic pain and, gastrointestinal problems. As a result, the child will experience several limitations in life and may need to be cared for either by the parent or care taker. Moreover, such child may require assistance in almost all of the activities of the daily living, such as bathing, feeding as well as assistance with turning, lifting the child whenever one wants to go out. One of the major problem faced by parents is attending to chronic health condition that the child might be suffering from. There is a great evidence that a child with cerebral palsy may also suffer from other illnesses, apart from the disability [2]. Thus, when compared to parents of typically developing children, parents of children with CP experience greater stress, lower psychological well-being, and worse physical health [3].

CP refers to a group of permanent disorders in the development of movement and posture, causing activity limitations, which are attributed to non-progressive disturbances that occurred in the developing fetal or infant brain [4]. The motor disturbance in a child with CP contributes to impaired cognitive ability, communication disorders, musculoskeletal problems, perception disturbance as well as epilepsy [3]. These problems associated with cerebral palsy may result in physical, social, psychological wellbeing and economic burden to the parents, families and community at large. The presence of a child with cerebral palsy in the family can be a source of great disappointment and stress to families. Significant number of research in this area has revealed the stress level endured by parents of children born with CP. The high stress levels among the parents were related to medical and social services that parents have to source during their predicament in raising a challenged child [2]. Mothers of children with CP are exposed to psychological pressure, are under the impact of stress and depression, and are worried for their child's future [5]. Most of their time is spend on the child's nutrition, health, treatment, rehabilitation and are subjected to financial burdens.

CP is an important example of a medical condition that requires competent, comprehensive, continuous, compassionate and community-based care [6]. Based on this, it is of utmost important to equip parents and their families with knowledge and skills to enable them to provide necessary support to their children. It is a permanent disorder that requires collective efforts from parents and health care providers such as occupational health therapist, speech and physical therapists. The health demands for a child with cerebral palsy may also place psychological, social and economic burden on parents and families. Therefore, it is also critical that primary care providers (PCP) be involved and knowledgeable about the current and future care plan for the best outcome for each child [6]. Parents, especially mothers are drivers of care, they do more work related to the care of a child. Caring for such a child who depends on care from others, can be energy draining, and mothers may require both social, psychological and financial support from other people to sustain their caring journey.

2. Effects of cerebral palsy

CP is a complex societal problem characterized, by social, psychological and economic implications requiring a collective multi-sectoral approach [2]. Parents often suffer from stress emanating from a number of factors; family members that feels taking care of a child with cerebral palsy is a waste of time and resources [6], financial strains that is incurred from medical expenses, transportation, nutrition, buying nappies as this child may spend the rest of her life in disposable nappies [5, 6] and many more. Despite all challenges endured by parents in caring for their children with CP, parents' attitude towards their children remains positive. They are optimistic about the condition of their children and also believe that physiotherapy is a beneficial intervention in the management of their children [3]. These hopes that parents have for their children is the driving force behind their existence.

2.1 Cerebral palsy and quality of parental life

Parenting a child requires considerable resources and time, but the demand for these resources may increase if the child to be cared for is mentally or physically challenged. To manage and cope with a child 's functional limitation and possible life- long dependence presents a multifaceted challenge for parents as well as the entire family [7]. Although some parents cope well with the additional demand of raising a child with CP, some studies showed that parents of such children experience tension and struggle especially the mothers who has to be with this child most of the time providing care. Mothers of such children are overwhelmed with the caring responsibilities, some of them left even their formal employment to stay home with their disabled children. Relinquishing one 's career may pause a significant setback to ones' life [8]. In some cases, mothers failed to take care of their own health and that of other siblings, thus affecting the physical and psychological health and, ultimately the quality of life of parents.

Caring for a child with CP may affect the quality of life for parents and families in many ways. Generally, parents of children with CP show high stress levels [2] and depression with ill-mental state compared to parents of children without disabilities. CP is a multifaceted disorder accompanied by several functional limitations. Although motor function is considered as the main challenge of CP, this developmental disorder is also accompanied by several limitations, such as sensory, communication and intellectual challenges [7]. Caring is a noble activity cherished by most of the mothers caring for young children in every community. This noble function may become a nightmare, when the child to be cared for is having functional limitations. Mothers of such children may go to an extent of diverting their focus from other important issues in the family and concentrate on the caregiving activities. Activities of the daily living may be overlooked, so as the other members in the family who might be depending on this caregiver for existence. This may however, results in high stress levels, anxiety and depression among caregivers.

Apart from the caregiving responsibilities, mothers of children with functional limitations are often challenged by chronic health- related problems that these children may experience in life. Several studies have affirmed that, most of the children born with CP usually suffers from one or two chronic conditions [2]. Thus, parents have to find means to respond to the health needs of the child with CP either through seeking for professional help from formal recognized health institutions or through home based therapies. Caring for a child with CP may affect the physical well- being, social well- being, freedom, independence of parents. The demands for caring for such a child has further created greater stress than the severity of the child 's disability, as it was revealed in one study, where parents with children born with CP felt that they were more disabled than the people there were caring for [9].

Parents of children with CP have lower quality of life which is associated with high levels of stress, anxiety and depression: The high stress level and depression is often associated with factors such as child's behavior, cognitive problems, low caregiver self-efficacy and low social support [7]. Therefore, due to the physical, psychological and social challenges that parents of children with CP usually experience, there should be an ongoing intervention like social, psychological and financial support to alleviate suffering among such parent.

2.2 Impact of cerebral palsy on family relationships

In the African context, family is a source of strength, and a shoulder to lean on during difficult times. Failure of the families to take up this extensive role has devastating effects on the lives of other members in the family. The family is a complex and interactive social system and each experience within family, affect every member. Components of the system continually change to keep it in balance. Within the family, there are three central subsystems: the spousal, parental, and sibling subsystems. In these three subsystems, marital relationship, is seen as a key factor in determining the quality of family life and core of the family unity. Raising a child with CP may be compounded if the parents of such children does not receive sufficient support within the family. Studies have shown that, living and caring for a child with CP can have a profound effect on parents- family, siblings and extended family relationships [10].

High stress levels, anger, depression that are evident in most families of children with CP are as a result of emotionally traumatized, broken family ties. Literature has shown that, the presence of a child with CP may have positive and negative influences on the relationships between families [2]. On the positive side, it can broaden horizons, increase family members' awareness of inner strength, enhance family bond and encourage networks to existing community groups [1], on the other hand, the physical, emotional demands and logistical complexities associated with raising a child with CP may have a negative effect on parents and families. Living with such a child can be a source of distress to families who might face several challenges to come to terms with the functional limitation of a child with CP.

2.2.1 A child with cerebral palsy and siblings

CP is a neurodevelopmental, irreversible and lifelong disorder that may have an impact on the life of families including siblings. It is important to understand the role of siblings towards raising a child with CP and what emotions do they feel towards this sibling with developmental disability. In normal families, older siblings play a facilitative role in cognitive and social development of younger siblings [11]. They also play a facilitative role in building a communicative competence among younger siblings whereby they play a role in stimulating language development. This facilitative role becomes a challenge should a child who is supposed to be mentored by older sibling is intellectually challenged. A significant number of older siblings of a child with CP, normally assumes the role of older siblings, regardless of their age, even the youngest sibling is able to take up such role. The ability of siblings to take up a caring role, depends on a number of factors, for example, the socio-economic status of families, the attitudes and expectations of parents and the severity of the disability [11] may affect the way the siblings react to the child with disability. Several studies reported that, the more severe the disability the more adversely affected the sibling of a child with CP [9].

Most of the powerful ties and human interactions are found between siblings as they act as surrogate parents, teachers and friends of children with CP. Thus, sibling relationships becomes very important in families, especially those living with physically or mentally challenged children. In main instances families of children with CP, do not receive emotional support when dealing with a child with CP. Literature has shown that, living with a child with CP involves tackling a wide range of challenges, such as physical, cognitive and behavioral [12]. Instead of engaging in activities such as socialization with others, participating in recreational activities, siblings of functionally challenged child devote most of their time in caring activities. Some suffers stigmatization by members of the society, calling them with names that relates to the child 's disability [2]. Bullying is another negative aspect that siblings of a child with CP face. Studies have indicated that siblings of physically or mentally challenged children are themselves a target for bullies [13]. They are teased of having a sibling with a developmental disorder.

In some families, the attention that parents gives to a child with CP, may create problems to other siblings as they may feel that their parents are neglecting them. This may result in increased stress levels, anxiety and depression among such siblings. Therefore, it's not a surprise that siblings who grow up with a sibling with CP tend to be a little more stressed when compared to children who do not live with someone with the disorder [13]. A study that was conducted in Ghana suggested that, the attitudes of siblings of children with CP need to be understood to ascertain ways to facilitate their acceptance in society as at times they face stigmatization as well as being sidelined by their own parents [14]. On a positive note, caring for a child with CP, may lead to increased maturity, sense of responsibility and tolerance among siblings [12, 14]. They're often more well-adjusted than their peers and more empathetic and caring towards people with special needs.

2.2.2 Cerebral palsy and marital relationships

High quality marital relationships in any marriage serve as a strong foundation of emotional and instrumental support. This support becomes more relevant and critical when parents in this relationship are faced with challenges of parenting a child with developmental disability and mostly CP. There is a growing evidence that, the stronger the bond between two parents of children with CP, the more the parents are likely to live a satisfying life [15] where they are able to support each other through thick and thin. Moreover, the high quality marital relationships may further reduce stress related ailments, thus promoting psychosocial wellbeing for both parents and a child with CP. Meanwhile, several studies have indicated that there is a strong association between high quality marital relationships and a considerate burden of living with a child with CP [15]. Parents with satisfying relationships normally experience less stress levels than those with troubled relationships. Although there are conflicting opinions from several authors who investigated the effects of disability on marital relationships, studies that compared marital relationships between parents of children with developmental disability and those of children without disabilities found that there was no significant difference in marital quality [16]. However, while some families of children with CP are free from stress and depression associated with parenting child with functional limitation, some families are challenged with the caring burden of living with a child with CP. The high stress levels among parents is believed to be associated to a number of factors i.e. caring burden as parents especially mothers have to renounce some of the activities of the daily living and concentrate more on the child with CP, medical expenses attached to parenting a child with CP, lack of social institutions that may incorporate the child with CP to the rest of the society and some reactions from members of the society who thinks raising a child with CP is a waste of time [2].

Given the indication that some children with CP often exhibit higher rates of behavioral problems than typically developing children, the relation of behavioral problems to parental wellbeing indicates that, interventions which address the child behavioral problems should be well-thought-out [1, 16]. The impact of a conflicting marriage on parental wellbeing should be well understood by trained professionals such as teacher and health care providers, who interacts with these families from time to time. Some literatures have revealed the act of blame especially among fathers of children with CP, where they are blaming mothers for being responsible for the child 's developmental disability [1]. This may however, result in high stress level and depression to the mother. The blame game can be a starting point of conflicting relationship which may result in divorce of such parents. Therefore, it is of utmost importance for professionals in the health sector to include parents, especially mothers when designing intervention for a child with CP as parents seems to be more affected than the people they are caring for [1, 17].

Studies that examined the influence of partner support on maternal stress and depression found that, mothers experienced high levels of stress when their child had cognitive impairment, even if partner support was high. These authors reiterated that, family functioning in families with a disabled child is better when the father is not directly implicated in caring for the child and mothers receive support from other people for the caring task [17]. The presence of spouse and their participation in the child's care provoked bitter feelings among mothers leading to parenting stress. Meanwhile, in some families, social support plays a significant role in minimizing parenting stress and improving life satisfaction [2]. Parenting stress is a negative psychological feeling associated with anxiety, frustration, and self-blame that can affect parenting behaviors and parenting functioning, while social support may be conceptualized as the provision of emotional, informational, and/or instrumental assistance that individuals receive from their social network [18]. There is a positive correlation between social support from families including spouse and parenting stress. Social support has been found to play an important mediating role in the association of several personal factors e.g. depression and emotional intelligence with life satisfaction [19]. The stronger the spousal relationship, the lesser the levels of stress will be among such parents, and this may eventually lead to life satisfaction.

2.3 Economic burden of cerebral palsy

The advancement in medical technology has increased the chances of children with CP to survive into adolescent and adulthood. However, this has led to the rise in the number of children with CP worldwide. Children with CP like other children with any form of disability requires an exceptional care with more cost implications. Although one might argue that, all children whether born with disability or not, often requires care with financial costs attached to it. Of course, all children require care with cost implication but the care and cost implications attached to a child born with CP or any other child with developmental disability is far much higher than that of other normal child. Documented studies have shown that the majority of families with children living with disabilities resulting from anomalies lives under severe poverty, remote from information and therefore not covered by the world statistics [20].

There is a growing evidence in the literature that parents of children with CP face unique financial challenges and meeting their child's needs and making financial ends meet is difficult for most of the parents. The management for CP includes various therapies, involving speech and physical therapy, as well as learning to use any sort of assistive device. In most cases, there is a need for the provision of special education at school and medication for some associated problems such as seizures, spasticity, and hearing or visual impairment. Apart from the costs related to health and education, children with CP also have specific needs related to basic care, some of children with CP need special diet for which the cost might be higher than the parents or family can afford. Most of the children with developmental disability or CP are bedridden which places another extra burden to parents and family, as this child may spent the rest of his life using disposable nappies [1]. Moreover, some children might need basic commodities such as special soaps and lotions, failure to use such commodities may lead to an extra health related condition and more financial implications.

Studies that investigated the economic burden on parents and family suggested that, countries that took a stance to provide financial assistance to children with disability should however, consider certain variables i.e. children with comorbidity and those without [21]. It is most likely, that parents of children with CP and comorbidity will have more financial burden than those without comorbidity, secondly, Older children require more financial assistance than younger children and government should streamline their budget on disability to ensure equity in distribution of such resources. Meanwhile, it is an unfortunate state that, even governments that provide financial assistance to people with disability have not addressed the state of affairs of children with disabilities properly, in most cases the governments decide what, how much and how often to provide to such children. Studies that assessed the financial burden of families of children CP found that, older children with CP required more financial assistance than normal children, and families with above average income could afford required minimal financial resources as it was found that they had no daily nursery expenses [21]. This shows that, there is in fact a necessity for need assessment to be carried out before countries attempt to assist parents of children with CP financially. The financial burden experienced by families of children with CP is less comprehensible to most governments. Therefore, evidence based information on the economic burden of CP, need to be available to assist policy makers in planning reasonable services and support for children with CP and other forms of disability.

Meanwhile, some studies have shown that children who experience limitations in daily activities require two to three times higher medical services than typical children [22], for example, a child with CP incurs a mean total average lifetime healthcare costs of US$22,143.00, whereas a child without any lifetime healthcare needs only incurs costs of US$1729.00, approximately 13 times lower [21]. Lifetime healthcare cost of a child with CP in South Korea was calculated to be US$26,383.00, which is 1.8 times the basic lifetime healthcare cost of the general population, US$14, 579.002. These healthcare needs lead to a higher cost of caring for children with CP as compared to children who are typically developing and the total cost often exceeds family's expectation [22]. Thus, children with developmental disability accompanied by comorbities.

3. Conclusion

CP is a lifelong problem that requires long term attention and care. The presence of a child with CP in any family can be a source of stress in any family and living with such a child may pose serious implications in terms of cost and social life to parents and families. The caring and economic burden endured by parents of children with CP has compromised immensely on the quality of life as it has affected the parents' psychological and physical wellbeing of parents and family. The consequences of caring and economic burden has an impact on the psychological and physical wellbeing of parents. This calls for well- designed interventions to support parents of children with CP.

Acknowledgements

The author would like to thank all authors of sources cited in this chapter. The information extracted from your writings contributed immensely to the completion of the chapter. I would like to state that, this work was not funded by any person nor organization.

Conflict of interest

No conflict of interest.

Notes/thanks/other declarations

I declare that, the information included in this chapter is my own work and all sources used are acknowledged in the reference list of the chapter.

Author details

Marian Sankombo
University of Namibia, Rundu, Namibia

*Address all correspondence to: msankombo@unam.na

References

[1] Sankombo MT. Experiences of parents with congenital abnormalities at Oshakati Intermediate hospital, Oshana region ([Mastersl thesis], University of Namibia)

[2] Al-Gamal E, Long T. Psychological distress and perceived support among Jordanian parents living with a child with cerebral palsy: A cross-sectional study. Scandinavian Journal of Caring Sciences. 2013;**27**(3):624-631

[3] Olawale OA, Deih AN, Yaadar RK. Psychological impact of cerebral palsy on families: The African perspective. Journal of Neurosciences in Rural Practice. 2013;**4**(2):159-163

[4] Glinac A, Matović L, Delalić A, Mešalić L. Quality of life in mothers of children with cerebral palsy. Acta Clinica Croatica. 2017;**56**(2):299-300

[5] Eker L, Tüzün EH. An evaluation of quality of life of mothers of children with cerebral palsy. Disability and Rehabilitation. 2004;**26**(23):1354-1359

[6] Gandhi RP, Klein U. Autism spectrum disorders: An update on oral health management. Journal of Evidence Based Dental Practice. 2014;**14**.115-126

[7] Ramanandi VH, Parmar TR, Panchal JK, Prabhakar MM. Impact of parenting a child with cerebral palsy on the quality of life of parents: A systematic review of literature. Disability, CBR & Inclusive Development. 2019;**30**(1):57-58

[8] Marian S, Magesa E, Fillipine N. Experiences of mothers of children born with celebral palsy in Oshana Region: Namibia. Global Journal of Health Science. 2020;**12**(1):1-72

[9] Cousino MK, Hazen RA. Parenting stress among caregivers of children with chronic illness: A systematic review. Journal of Pediatric Psychology. 2013;**38**(8):809-828

[10] Reichman NE, Corman H, Noonan K. Impact of child disability on the family. Maternal and Child Health Journal. 2008;**12**(6):679-683

[11] Mophosho M, Widdows J, Gomez MT. Relationships between adolescent children and their siblings with cerebral palsy: A pilot study. Journal on Developmental Disabilities. 2009;**15**(3):81

[12] Freeborn D, Knafl K. Growing up with cerebral palsy: Perceptions of the influence of family. Child: Care, Health and Development. 2014;**40**(5):671-679

[13] Martirosyan A. Sibling relationships in families with a child with special needs. A case study of a Norwegian family with a child with down syndrome and her three siblings [Master's thesis]

[14] Hartley SL, Seltzer MM, Barker ET, Greenberg JS. Marital quality and families of children with developmental disabilities. International Review of Research in Developmental Disabilities. 2011;**1**(41):1-29

[15] Karadeniz G, Balkan İ, Gazioğlu N, Duman N, Elmas E, Eyrenci A, et al. Marital adjustment among parents of children with developmental disabilities. Psychology-Traditions and Perspectives. 2015;**1**:161-168

[16] Risdal D, Singer GH. Marital adjustment in parents of children with disabilities: A historical review and meta-analysis. Research and Practice

for Persons with Severe Disabilities. 2004;**29**(2):95-103

[17] Pousada M, Guillamón N, Hernández-Encuentra E, Muñoz E, Redolar D, Boixadós M, et al. Impact of caring for a child with cerebral palsy on the quality of life of parents: A systematic review of the literature. Journal of Developmental and Physical Disabilities. 2013;**25**(5):545-577

[18] Wang Y, Huang Z, Kong F. Parenting stress and life satisfaction in mothers of children with cerebral palsy: The mediating effect of social support. Journal of Health Psychology. 2020;**25**(3):416-425

[19] Chen W, Zhang D, Pan Y, Hu T, Liu G, Luo S. Perceived social support and self-esteem as mediators of the relationship between parental attachment and life satisfaction among Chinese adolescents. Personality and Individual Differences. 2017;**108**:98-102

[20] Umar UI, Adamu H, Abdulkareem A. Economic evaluation of cerebral palsy in a resource-challenged setting. Nigerian Journal of Basic and Clinical Sciences [serial online] 2020 [cited 2022 Jun 23];**17**:50-56. Available from: https://www.njbcs.net/text.asp?2020/17/1/50/285471

[21] Kamaralzaman S, Ying TC, Mohamed S, Toran H, Satari N, Abdullah N. The economic burden of families of children with cerebral palsy in Malaysia. Malaysian Journal of Public Health Medicine. 2018;**2018**(Special 1):156-165

[22] Newacheck PW, Hughes DC, Stoddard JJ, Halfon N. Children with chronic illness and Medicaid managed care. Pediatrics. 1994;**93**(3):497-500

Chapter 6

Access to Healthcare Services Among Children with Cerebral Palsy in the Greater Accra Region of Ghana

Nathaniel Larbi Andah

Abstract

Children with cerebral palsy have quite a lot of challenges in accessing health care than those without disabilities. The purpose of the study was to explore the factors that influence parents in accessing healthcare services for their children with cerebral palsy. This study used a qualitative cross-sectional design using phenomenology. A total of 15 participants comprising parents of children with disabilities and healthcare providers provided data through in-depth interviews following written informed consent. Fifteen in-depth interviews were conducted. The interviews were recorded digitally and transcribed verbatim. Thematic analysis was adopted in the analysis of the data using Nvivo 12. Fifteen IDIs were completed: 10 parents of children with cerebral palsy and 5 healthcare providers. The study findings revealed individual factors such as transportation cost, distance to a health facility, and stigmatization as well as healthcare factors such as availability of specialized services, the attitude of health professionals, the physical environment of hospitals, and the availability of rehabilitation specialists influence parents access to healthcare services for their children with cerebral palsy. Access to healthcare services for children with cerebral palsy is influenced by individual factors (parental) and healthcare factors.

Keywords: cerebral palsy, healthcare services, access

1. Introduction

The World Disability report shows that approximately 15% of the global population are people with disabilities making them the largest minority group in the world [1]. WHO estimated that nearly 3% of the global population has cerebral palsy (CP) [2]. According to Janzek-hawlat [3] persons with CP experience discrimination in healthcare more than the general population. The Convention on the Right of Persons with Disabilities (CRPD) affirms that persons with disabilities have the right to achieve their highest standard of health care, without any discrimination [4]. However, the health care needs of children with CP are poor, particularly in low- and middle-income countries. In Africa, parents of children with CP experience social isolation from family, friends, and community members, discrimination from peers, transportation problem, and a financial challenge because of unemployment [5]. Aside from these challenges, parents of children with CP also experience challenges with the healthcare system including lack of provision of assistive devices, attitudes of healthcare professionals, and high cost of healthcare services [5]. In Ghana, parents of children with CP also face similar challenges in accessing health facilities, these are due to inaccessible environment, distance to a health facility, transportation, discriminatory attitudes of health workers, neglect, stigmatization, and inadequate healthcare services [6–9].

Access to healthcare is a development issue, as well as a question of the realization of rights. A significant focus of Sustainable Development Goal 3 "Good Health and Well-being" is to advance access to healthcare services for All through the behavior accomplishment of Universal Health Coverage (UHC) [10]. Despite this, children with CP experience financial, structural, and social problems in accessing healthcare services [11]. According to WHO [2] children with CP usually do not benefit from health promotion and prevention programs because they are scarcely targeted. This study is therefore designed to employ qualitative design using phenomenology to identify the factors that influence access to healthcare services for children with CP in the Greater Accra Region of Ghana.

2. Methods

2.1 Research design

The study used a qualitative cross-sectional design using phenomenology to assess the knowledge of parents of children with CP on National Health Policy, explore the perceptions of parents of children with CP on the implementation of the National Health Policy in Ghana, identify parental factors and healthcare factors that influence access to healthcare services for children with CP. Phenomenology allows participants to share their perceptions, feelings, and lived experiences in accessing healthcare services for their wards with CP and how these experiences influence their ability to access healthcare for their children with CP.

2.2 Study area

The study was conducted in the Greater Accra Region (GAR) of Ghana because there are quite a lot of parents of children with CP and an existing self-help group (**Figure 1**). There are over 500 parents of children with CP and about 20 existing self-help groups in GAR. The study considered the Special Mothers Project self-help group in Okponglo in the Greater Accra Region. The Special Mothers Project has been existing for the past 7 years and is open to every parent of children with disabilities especially those with children with cerebral palsy. GAR is the capital town of Ghana and has the smallest area of Ghana's sixteen (16) administrative regions. GAR can be found in the South-East part of the country and it is surrounded on the north by the Eastern Region, on the east by the Volta Region, on the south by the Gulf of Guinea, and on the west by the Central Region. GAR is divided into sixteen districts and its political administration is through the local government. Each district is administered by a Chief Executive who represents the central government.

DOI: http://dx.doi.org/10.5772/intechopen.106684

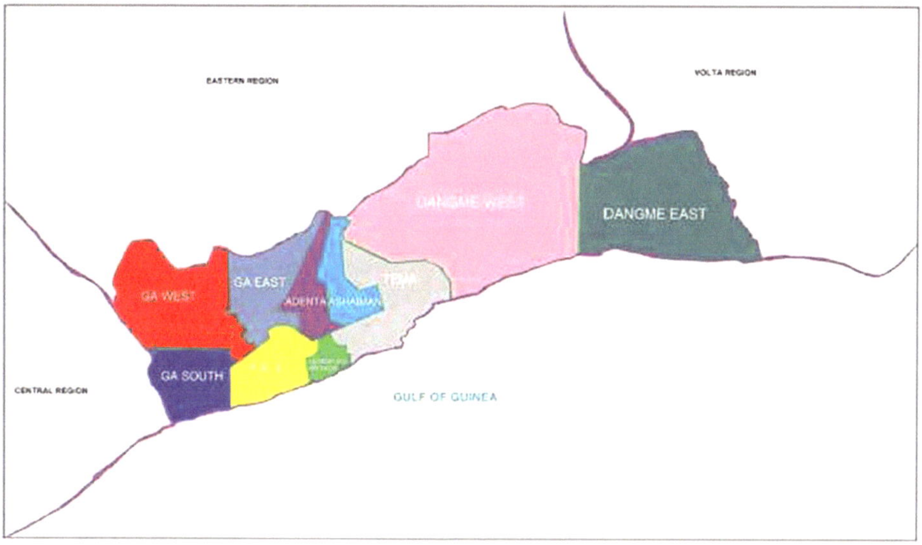

Figure 1.
Map showing health districts in Greater Accra. Source: Google Maps [12].

2.3 Study participants

The study participants were parents of children with CP between the ages of 3 to 17 years who attend a special school in the Greater Accra Region, this is because 17% of children are diagnosed with CP within the age range and healthcare providers who provide services to children with CP within the study period will be part of the study (**Table 1**).

2.4 Selection of study participants

The respondents for this study were recruited using a purposive sampling technique. This sampling technique is a non-probability sampling used to select participants based on the experiences and characteristics they possess that best fit for the study. The inclusion and exclusion criteria were considered in selecting the participants for the study. Parents of children with CP who met the inclusion criteria were purposively sampled at home for an interview in the study. Three (3) participants were selected each day for the in-depth interview (IDI) while the key informant interview (KII) was also used for healthcare workers who met the inclusion criteria until the point of saturation was reached. Saturation was determined when no new information was emerging from the study participants. A total of fifteen (15) participants reached saturation, including 10 parents of children with CP and 5 health care providers. The study purposefully identified and selected ten (10) children with CP who are eligible for the study at the school level based on age, sex, and disability and proceeded to their homes to consent to their parents or caregivers for recruitment for an in-depth interview.

Also, five (5) health facilities both private and public in the Greater Accra Region were selected for key informant interviews based on specialized and generalized healthcare services provided. Five (5) eligible healthcare providers within the selected health facilities who directly offer healthcare services to children with CP were

Characteristics of Participants	Number of Participants	
	Parents for IDIs	Healthcare providers for KIIs
Special schools		
Woodfield Manor Special School	5	—
Dzorwulu Special School	5	—
Health Facility		
Cocoa Clinic (Private)	—	1
Alpha Medical Center (Private)	—	1
La General Hospital (Public)	—	1
Achimota Hospital (Public)	—	1
Kaneshie (Public)	—	1
Sex		
Male	1	3
Female	9	2
Age (years)	**Children with CP**	
3–10	10	
11–17	5	
20–29	1	
30–39	7	4
40+	2	1
Educational Level		
No Formal Education	—	—
Primary	1	
JHS/SHS	6	
Tertiary	3	5
Religion		
Christianity	9	5
Islam	1	
Occupation		
Trader	5	
Teacher	3	
Student/Unemployed	2	
Occupational Therapist		2
Physiotherapist		2
General Health Practitioner		1
Marital Status		
Single	6	4
Married	4	1

Table 1.
Socio-demographic characteristics of participants.

purposively selected for the study based on a particular set of characteristics such as experience, skills, knowledge, and highest educational level for a KII. This is to get an adequate number of participants for the study.

2.5 Data collection methods

The study used both IDIs and KIIs to collect primary data from study participants. IDIs were steered within the homes of identified parents of children with CP at their convenience. Also, all KIIs were steered within the work premises of the identified healthcare provider upon appointment. The IDIs and KIIs were directed by an interview guide containing questions and probes that directed the interviewer.

2.6 Selection of study participants

The respondents for this study were recruited using a purposive sampling technique. This sampling technique is a non-probability sampling used to select participants based on the experiences and characteristics they possess that best fit for the study. The inclusion and exclusion criteria were considered in selecting the participants for the study. Parents of children with CP who met the inclusion criteria were purposively sampled at home for an interview in the study. Three (3) participants were selected each day for the IDI while the KII was also used for healthcare workers who met the inclusion criteria until the point of saturation was reached. Saturation was determined when no new information was emerging from the study participants. A total of fifteen (15) participants reached saturation, including 10 parents of children with CP and 5 health care providers. The study purposefully identified and selected ten (10) children with CP who are eligible for the study at the school level based on age, sex, and disability and proceeding to their homes to consent to their parents or caregivers for recruitment for IDIs. Also, five (5) health facilities both private and public in the Greater Accra Region were selected for KII based on specialized and generalized healthcare services provided.

2.7 Data collection tools

An interview guide, a field notebook, a voice recorder, and a field diary were used to collect data during the study. The interview guide for both IDIs and KIIs contained questions and probes on; the knowledge of parents on the Persons with Disability Act of Ghana, NHIS, perceptions of parents about the implementation of the National Health Policy in Ghana, parental factors in accessing health care, healthcare factors (challenges), and specialized services available for children with CP. Both in-depth interviews and key informant interviews were recorded using a voice recorder and field diary to take key notes found on the field.

2.8 Data analysis

All IDIs and KIIs were recorded with the participants' permission. Interviews conducted in the local dialect were transcribed literally into English by the research assistant who was conversant with the language. All transcriptions were confirmed and transported into Nvivo version 12. The coding of themes was developed thematically in line with the objectives of the study and emerging themes in the field. The inductive and deductive approaches were used in the coding process. Themes were summarized into appropriate sub-headings using queries. A codebook was developed for themes that will emerge during interviews on the field and appropriate excerpts were used to support the theme.

3. Results

3.1 Knowledge of National health policy in Ghana

The study revealed that the majority of the participants had a fair knowledge of the National Health Policy in Ghana, and explained it as a policy that aims to promote health for everyone in Ghana. Some participants also explained the National Health Policy according to their understanding of health in the Persons with Disability Act (Act 715) and the NHIS in Ghana (**Table 2**). The participants were therefore asked about their knowledge of health in the Persons with Disability Act. The participants described health in the Persons with Disability Act as a means of getting access to healthcare services without any barriers and discrimination. Participants believed that the health in Persons with Disability Act means having access to healthcare services without any discrimination, physical and attitudinal barriers as well as accessing free specialized services in the public health facilities (**Figure 2**). The belief of having access to healthcare services without any barrier was universal among the participants. Those who hold these beliefs also indicated that the persons with disability act mandate the State to provide financial support to persons with disabilities. The study showed that the participants were knowledgeable about the NHIS. The respondents emphasized how the NHIS serves as a safety net and has replaced the cash-and-carry system of service delivery. Some of the respondents also attributed the NHIS as the means of ensuring sustainable financing for health.

3.2 Perception of the implementation of the National health policy in Ghana

The study findings showed that participants agreed on the implementation of the National Health Policy of Ghana. Participants were asked questions about their perception of health in the implementation of the Persons with Disability Act and on the NHIS (NHIS). Some of the perceptions revealed in this study were the ineffectiveness of the Persons with Disability Act, poor quality health service, and less health service coverage by the NHIS. It also showed that participants were unanimous on the health service coverage by the NHIS. All participants acknowledged that the NHIS does cover some aspects of healthcare services like consultation fee, patient card, half of the lap fees, part of medication, and one-month cost of physiotherapy but does not cover tertiary services like surgery and some specialized services like speech and language therapy, occupational therapy among others. Participants revealed in the study that these tertiary and specialized services are constantly needed by children with CP.

3.3 Parental factors

The choices made by parents as to whether to seek healthcare for their children with CP is dependent on other factors. According to Khatri and Karkee [14], parental factors are more likely to shape the health-seeking behavior of individuals. Study participants were therefore asked questions on parental factors that can influence access

Concepts	Operational definitions
1. Approachability/Accommodation	The extent to which health care services are provided in different ways to meet the health needs of clients irrespective of barriers.
2. Acceptability	The level of comfort existing between client and provider with fixed characteristics including sex, age, race, ethnicity among others.
3. Affordability	The relationship between providers charges and the client's ability to pay for services; Cost of service covered by health insurance and client's ability to pay the amount left.
4. Appropriateness	The ability of health providers to properly use health services, products, and resources for the benefit of clients.
5. Availability	Provider's ability to have all the required resources needed to meet the client's health needs.

Source: [13].

Table 2.
Dimensions of access to health care services.

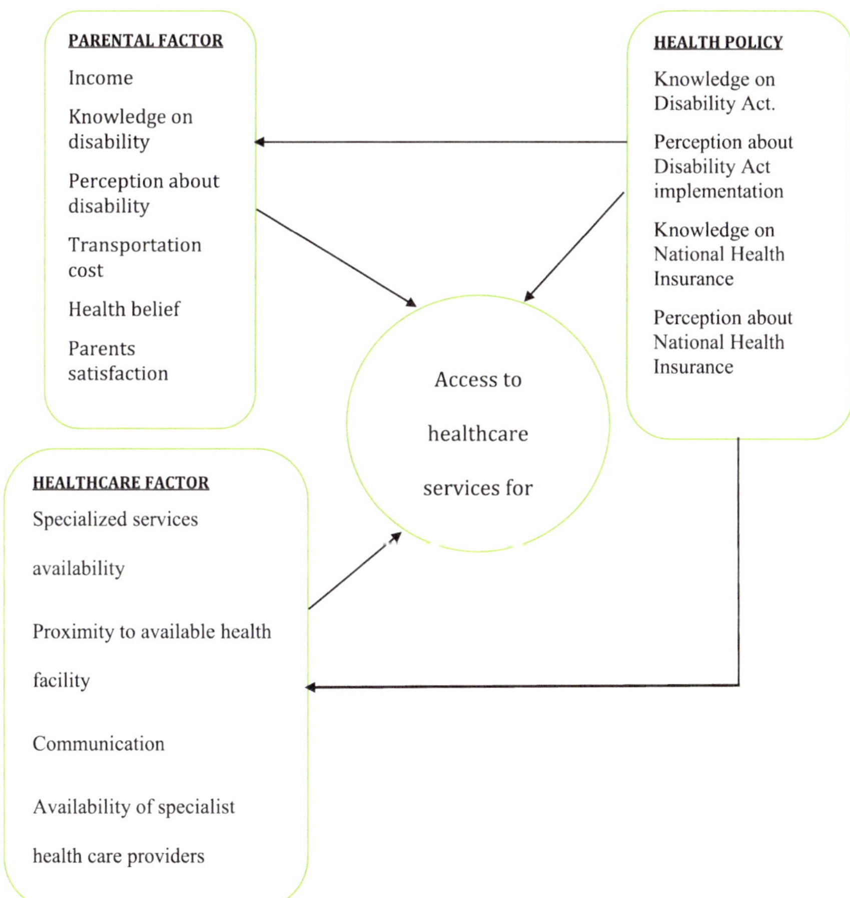

Figure 2.
Conceptual framework- Factors influencing access to healthcare (Adapted from the WHO; International classification of functioning, disability, and health [8, 9].

to healthcare services for children with CP. From the study findings, participants mentioned knowledge of disability, perception about disability (CP), income spent on child's health care, transportation cost, and satisfaction as factors that influence access to healthcare services for children with CP (**Figure 2**).

3.3.1 Causes of disability

Concerning knowledge of the causes of disability, some participants attributed it to spirituality, brain damage (medical condition), and diseases. Some participants believe that haters from families can make a child have a disability through witchcraft and voodoo especially when the child has a bright future. The study revealed that parents with such beliefs do not seek medical care for their children but rather seek spiritual healing for their children with CP.

3.3.2 Symptoms of CP

Regarding the signs and symptoms of CP, the following were mentioned: poor eye contact, poor posture, and balance, communication, as well as impaired fine and gross motor function.

3.3.3 Treatment

Considering treatment, the majority of the respondents believed that CP cannot be treated (cured) but can be managed through the following means: Specialized healthcare services including physiotherapy, occupational therapy, speech and language therapy, and generalized healthcare services including primary healthcare like screening and health checkups. The majority of the respondents with this knowledge seek healthcare for their children with CP as revealed in this study.

3.3.4 Perceptions of disability

The results of the study also revealed that respondents share different perceptions of disability. Some of the respondents mentioned that disability can result in stigmatization, discrimination disrespect, loneliness, depression, and even suicide. Respondents agreed that when someone has a disability stigmatization and discrimination inevitably lead to depression, loneliness, and suicidal ideation. The study showed that respondents with such perceptions feel reluctant to seek healthcare for their wards with CP with the fear of being stigmatized and discriminated against. Some participants also mentioned that disability can be frustrating and lead to the loss of a job.

Participants believed that negative perception about disability may lead to less access to healthcare services for children with CP while the positive perception may lead to frequent access to healthcare services. Respondents with a negative perception of disability do not seek regular healthcare for their children with CP but rather go to seek spiritual healing for their wards with CP. Also, it was revealed that respondents with positive perceptions frequently seek healthcare for their children with CP.

3.3.5 The financial burden on a child with CP health care

The study showed that the majority of the respondents are not able to access healthcare for their wards with CP as they spend a greater part of their income on their child's health. Participants agreed that the healthcare needs of children with CP are a lot and most expensive. They stated that specialized services like physiotherapy, occupational therapy, speech and language therapy, and special nutrition help to manage children with CP but these services are expensive and sometimes they find it difficult to access (**Figure 2**). However, some participants also specified that because of the expensive nature of specialized services they tend to do basic physiotherapy for their wards in their homes since they cannot keep up with the services in the hospitals. Participants were unanimous on how they spend so much money on both primary and secondary healthcare services for their children with CP and this discourages them from accessing healthcare services for their children with CP. Parents of children with CP all agreed that income level may influence access to healthcare services in either a positive or negative way depending on the kind of job a parent has (**Table 2**). The study revealed that access to healthcare services for children with CP is higher among parents with a higher income than those with a lower income. Some participants also stated that the kind of job one does determine the level of income.

3.4 Transportation

The study revealed that parents of children with CP do experience transportation problems and that discourages them from accessing healthcare services for their children with CP. All participants agreed that transportation is another factor that influences access to healthcare services. The majority of the participants stated that their means of transportation to the hospital is public transport (trotro, taxi, uber). All participants mentioned that transportation problems include access to public transport, transportation cost, and stigmatization in public transport.

Concerning access to public transport majority of the respondents agreed that most public transport designs are not accessible and friendly to children with CP. This makes it difficult for them to access public transport to a health facility. It was also revealed in this study that all respondents agreed there is no designated space for persons with disabilities inside public transport. This makes them feel very uncomfortable when using public transport to a health facility. Findings from this study showed that respondents who use public transport do not frequently access healthcare services for their children with CP as they are discouraged from all the hustle and frustration, they face from accessing public transport.

Some of the participants asserted that transportation cost to the closest health facility is expensive and, in most cases, uber or taxi drivers do not want to render services to them due to their children with disabilities. Participants also believed that commercial drivers (uber and taxi) charge them a higher cost because of their children with disabilities. The study found that passengers, conductors (mate), and commercial drivers (trotro) do stigmatize parents of children with CP when boarding a car to a health facility. Study participants specified that passengers do not want to sit by them with the belief that they will end up having a child with a disability and also bus conductors (mate) and commercial drivers (trotro) also ask them to pay for the entire seat or else they will not pick them up. This discourages parents from accessing healthcare for their children with CP.

Also, some respondents mentioned that stigmatization from passengers, bus conductors, and drivers do put them off sometimes and not access healthcare for their child with CP.

3.4.1 Satisfaction

The results of the study showed that participants agreed that satisfaction with health care services does influence their access to healthcare. The participants attributed satisfaction to quality health care, waiting time for treatment, and cost-effectiveness of healthcare services. Respondents explained quality health care as the one that is considered to be safe, efficient, inclusive, patient-centered, timely, and that makes customers happy. Respondent also believed that when patients do not get quality healthcare, they may reduce the number of times they visit a particular health facility or they may stop accessing health care from those particular health facilities.

3.5 Identification of health service needs (health care factors)

From the study findings, participants were generally able to identify healthcare factors that include specialized services availability, proximity to an available health facility, availability of specialist healthcare providers, accessibility of building and equipment, and healthcare provider's attitude do influence access to healthcare services for children with CP (**Figure 2**).

3.5.1 Availability of specialized services

Respondents mentioned some specialized services that health facilities need to make available for children with CP, these include speech and language therapy, physiotherapy, occupational therapy, behavioral therapy, augmentative communication, and dietary approaches. Respondents believed that these specialized services help children with talking, walking, participating in the activities of daily life (such as brushing teeth and getting dressed), interacting with others, learning social skills, and managing their emotions. Study participants mentioned that they feel encouraged to access health care from health facilities that provide specialized services.

3.5.2 Proximity to an available health facility

All study participants mentioned that distance from a patient's (clients) home to the nearest health facility can influence access to health care. Participants believed that clients are discouraged to access the closest health facility when they face a transportation problem and have to travel far distances. However, clients whose home is not too far from the nearest hospital is encouraged to access healthcare for their child with CP.

3.5.3 Availability of specialist healthcare providers

From the study findings, participants acknowledged and stated that the availability of rehabilitation specialists in health centers influences their access to healthcare for their children with CP. Respondents asserted that some hospitals have specialized services written on their signboards but do not provide such services because specialists are scarce. This influences their decision to access healthcare services from certain health facilities. Respondents believed that rehabilitation specialists like physiotherapists, speech and language therapists, and occupational therapists are very few and scarce in Ghana, especially in the rural areas. Respondents also asserted that they have to travel long distances to access these specialized services in the urban centers which sometimes transportation cost and rehabilitation cost becomes a challenge to them.

Accommodations	Suggested approaches
Using features of universal design equipment	Height-adjustable examination tables, seated scales, accessible wheelchair diagnostic equipment including mammography equipment
Structural modification of facilities	Configuring the layout of clinical examination rooms, installing ramps and grab rails, ensuring barrier-free path from transit to the clinic, widening doorways, installing lifts, modifying washrooms (toilet and urinal), providing adaptable seats for those who cannot stand.
Communicating health information in appropriate formats	A health care provider can provide health information in large prints, braille, picture format, audio, or even in the video; speaking clearly and slowly to clients to ensure understanding, providing sign language interpreting services.
Using alternative models to deliver health service	Using mobile clinic services, telemedicine, assistance with transportation to a health facility.

Table 3.
Reasonable accommodation and suggested approaches.

3.5.4 Accessibility of building and equipment

Study participants agreed that many health centers are not disability-friendly. They linked the accessibility of the building to the physical environment of the health facility including entrance to consulting rooms, OPD, and top floors. Some participants also stated that equipment like standing frames, power tables, parallel bars, and stand-assist devices in most hospitals are not friendly to children with CP (**Table 3**). Participants believed that most rehabilitation equipment in certain hospitals is meant for stroke patients and not for children with CP.

3.5.5 Healthcare providers attitude

Attitudes of healthcare providers play a significant role in parents' decisions to access health care for their children with disabilities. Some participants acknowledged the fact that not all healthcare providers' attitude is bad. However, the majority of the respondents stated that their experience with healthcare providers has been bad and that discourages them from accessing healthcare for their children with CP. It was strongly perceived that bad behavior like discrimination from healthcare providers towards parents of children with CP would rather discourage them from accessing health care.

4. Discussion

4.1 Knowledge of National health policy

The level of knowledge of the National Health Policy was well known among almost all the participants as it was considered a policy that aims to promote health for everyone in Ghana. This view is similar to Vartan and Montuschi's [15]'s assertion that the national health policy has been developed to promote, restore, and maintain good health for all people living in Ghana. Participants also explained their knowledge of the national health policy from the persons with disabilities Act perspective as a means of getting access to healthcare services without any barrier or discrimination. This finding in this study is consistent with the Americans with Disability Act (1990) Section 504 of the Rehabilitation Act that forbids discrimination based on disability and also the Person with Disability Act (2006) of Ghana Section 4 (1) and (6) that prohibit discriminate, exploit or to subject a person with disabilities to abusive or degrading treatment.

The present study findings indicate that the majority of the respondents had sufficient knowledge regarding the NHIS (NHIS) describing it as a safety net that replaces the cash and system of service delivery in Ghana. This finding is in agreement with a study conducted by Akande and Akande [16] on "The Awareness and Attitude of Practitioners on NHIS in Llorin showed that all respondents were aware of the scheme but only a few did not know. Another study conducted by Dixon et al. [17] on "Ghana's NHIS: a national level investigation of members' perceptions on service provision in Ghana" found that the NHIS replaces cash-and-carry, which required individuals to make a payment from their pockets at service usage. However, another study by Gopalan and Durairaj [18] showed that better-educated individuals can access diverse sources of information, correctly process and take advantage of benefits than those who are less educated and those without formal education. Those who could not afford to spend more on the healthcare needs of children with CP may adopt other coping mechanisms such as alternative care, presenting late at the health facilities, or not receiving care at all.

4.2 Perception of implementation of National health policy

Findings from this current study revealed that respondents are influenced in accessing health care for their wards even when they are insured as they perceived the implementation of the National Health Policy to be ineffective concerning poor-quality health service for the insured. This finding is similar to Bruce et al. [19] study results on "The perceptions and experiences of health care providers and clients in two districts in Ghana" which showed that insured clients are not satisfied with the healthcare they received and perceived that they were given poorer quality services and tend to wait longer as compared to those making Out of Pocket Payment (OOP). The present study also revealed that the implementation of the National Health Policy is ineffective as respondents perceived that it does not cover major specialized services and treatment for children with CP. This study finding is in contrast to Dalinjog and Laar's [20] study on "The effectiveness of the National Health Policy in Ghana" which found that both insured and uninsured respondents had positive perceptions and were satisfied with the care provided.

4.3 Parental factors

The study discovered that participants were generally aware of some of the factors that influence access to healthcare services among children with CP. A study conducted by Khartri and Karkee [14] showed that distance to health facilities, social support, age, the behavior of health workers, and access to quality health services shapes how parents access healthcare for their children and themselves. This finding is in agreement with Boz et al. [21] study on "The affecting factors of healthcare services demand in terms of health services use: A field application in Edirne city" found that personal income, gender, attitudes, and behaviors of physicians affect access to healthy demand. In the same study, it was reported that family members, perception of economic level, attitudes, and behaviors of physicians were found to influence health demand. Findings from this current study revealed that participants know about disability regarding the causes, signs, and symptoms as well as treatment for children with CP. This positively influenced parents' access to healthcare for their children with CP. This finding is consistent with Matt's [22] study on "Perception of disability among caregivers of children with disabilities in Nicaragua" which found that parents with higher education have a better understanding and knowledge of their children's disability and frequently access health care services for their wards than parents with lower or no education. The current study findings also agree with Khatri and Karkee's [14] assertion that illiterate parents who belong to the lowest wealth quintile have lower access and use of healthcare for their children with CP.

Also, considering the causes of disability, this current study revealed that respondents know the causes of disability. Findings from the study showed that disability can be caused by disease and neurological problems leading to brain damage. This finding is in agreement with the Center for Diseases Control and Prevention [23] assertion that risk factors such as infections during pregnancy, premature birth, and diseases like jaundice can cause CP.

Respondents in this study linked signs and symptoms of CP to poor eye contact, poor posture and balance, communication difficulties, and impaired fine and gross motor function. This finding agrees with the CP Alliance [24] assertion that children with CP show signs and symptoms like swallowing difficulties, poor muscle spasms, low muscle tone, poor muscle control, reflexes, and posture, drooling, developmental delay, gastrointestinal problems, and not walking by 12–18 months. It was found from this study that treatment for children with CP includes physiotherapy, occupational therapy, and speech and language therapy. This finding is consistent with the CP Guide [25] statement that children with CP can improve their motor skills with alternative therapy, medication, and surgery through multidisciplinary teams such as neurologists, orthopedic surgeons, developmental pediatricians, physiotherapists, occupational therapists, nutritionists, respiratory therapists, psychologists to assess ability and behavior and speech and language, therapist.

It was also found in this study that perceptions of parents about their children's disability (CP) also influence their decision to access healthcare for their children with CP. It was also established that stigmatization, discrimination, disrespect, loneliness, depression, and suicidal ideation are linked to disability (CP). This is similar to Physioplus's [26] assertion that families with a child with a disability are more prone to depression, suicide, financial problem, relationship challenges, divorce, and bankruptcy. This statement is also in line with another study by Butchner [27] on "society's attitude towards persons with disabilities" which found that society perceives that disability is a curse and punishment from ancestors and gods. Also, Duran and Ergun [28] in their study on "The stigma perceived by parents of children with disability: an interpretative phenomenological analysis study in Balikesir found that the majority of people often have negative perceptions and stigmatizing attitudes towards children with disabilities (CP) and their families. In the same study, it was found that parents of children with disabilities cope with insults and rude behaviors from community members while they struggle with the challenges of their children with CP. This is similar to a previous study by Opoku et al. [6] who affirmed that persons with disabilities are severely stigmatized, discriminated against, and excluded from all forms of the development process resulting in limiting their opportunities to be engaged in decision-making and accessing healthcare.

Income was found from this current study to influence parents' access to health care services for their children with CP. Respondents emphasized that the level of income of a parent is dependent on the kind of job the parent does. This present study revealed that parents of children with CP who have no jobs find it difficult to access healthcare services for their wards due to the cost of treatment. This finding is in line with DeVoe et al. [29] assertion that children with CP from lower-income families experience more gaps in healthcare than children with CP from higher-income families.

Moreover, this study discovered that transportation is another factor that influences access to health care. Findings from this study indicated that transportation cost, distance to the nearest health facility, and stigmatization from drivers, passengers, and bus conductors (mate) influence respondents' ability to access healthcare services for their children with CP. A previous study showed that healthcare utilization is influenced by the direct costs of healthcare services, travel time, and patient income [30]. This is in line with another study conducted by Bulamu Healthcare [31] in Uganda which specified that patients complain about poor sanitation, lack of drugs and equipment, long waiting times, rude behavior of health workers, and poor referrals. However. in that same study it was revealed that over 8000 rural Ugandans travel as far as 50 miles to attend a Bulamu weeklong medical camp for healthcare.

Also, findings from this present study showed that respondents are not satisfied with the waiting time and cost of health care services. Respondents from this present study linked healthcare satisfaction to quality health care, waiting time for treatment, and cost-effectiveness of healthcare services. This assertion is consistent with Khatri and Karkee's [14] statement that quality health care accounts for patient satisfaction especially in terms of waiting time, cost of service, coordination, information, and physician's behavior. This finding agrees with Janzek-hawlat's [3] findings that some physicians in public health facilities can be very rude due to the workload mounted on them.

4.4 Healthcare factors

Considering specialized services available, the present study found that respondents were informed about the available specialized services for their children with CP. It was discovered that speech and language therapy, physiotherapy, occupational therapy, behavioral therapy, augmentative communication, and dietary were some of the specialized services available but scarce and that makes it difficult to access healthcare for their children due to waiting time for treatment. Respondents in this present study believed that children who can access these services will be able to walk, interact with others through play, learn social skills, seat properly, and have good muscle and neck control as well as good balance and body posture. This finding agrees with Balcı's [32] study on "Current Rehabilitation Methods for Cerebral Palsy" which found that children with CP that undergo muscle strengthening training, manual stretching, massage, neurodevelopmental treatment, conductive education, speech and language therapy, occupational therapy, and dieting have good body posture, balancing, neck coordination, strong muscle control and can walk sometimes. However, the lack of appropriate services for individuals with CP is a significant barrier to health care. For instance, qualitative research in Uttar Pradesh and Tamil Nadu states of India revealed that after the cost, the lack of services in the area was the second most significant barrier to using health facilities [8, 9].

Also, it was found from this current study that proximity to an available health facility is another factor that influences access to healthcare for children with CP. From the study, respondents were discouraged to access the nearest health facility when transportation and distance to the health facility are problems. This finding is similar to Awoyemi et al. [33] study on "Effect of Distance on Utilization of Health Care Services in Rural Kogi State in Nigeria" which found that distance and total cost of healthcare affects the utilization of both public and private hospitals. This finding also agrees with Nesbitt et al. [34] study on "Barriers and facilitating factors in access to health services in the Republic of Moldova" which found that distance from a health service provider, travel time, and waiting time to see a health professional is are strong factors that influence access to health care.

Moreover, the availability of specialists in hospitals was found in this present study to be scarce in most hospitals, and because of that, only a few respondents travel a long distance to access these specialized services for their wards. This finding is consistent with WHO [35] reported that the registered number of rehabilitation specialists is far below the required minimum of 750 per 1 million even in developed countries. In addition to this, the present study revealed that most public and private hospitals are not environmentally friendly for children with CP who use wheelchairs. Respondents asserted that most public hospitals do not have elevators and ramps making it difficult to access healthcare services for their wards. This finding is in line with Jamshidi et al. [36] study on "The effects of environmental factors on the patients' outcomes in hospital environments: A review of the literature" found that medical equipment adaptability, unit layout, room features, ramps, and elevators affect patients' access to healthcare. Another study by Douglas and Douglas, [37] revealed that patients' need for personal space, a homely welcoming atmosphere, a supportive environment, ramps, and elevators influence access to their healthcare. Cristina and Candidate [11] also found in their study that out of 256 respondents, 9 (4%) were not able to access the building and 47(18%) were not able to be transferred from their wheelchair to the examination table.

It was also found from this study that some healthcare providers discriminate against parents of children with CP when seeking primary healthcare services and physiotherapy. This finding agrees with the WHO [8, 9] report that parents of children with disabilities face stigmatization and discrimination in most health facilities. This finding is also in line with Rogers et al. [38] study on "Discrimination in healthcare settings is associated with disability in Older Adults: Health and Retirement Study, 2008-2012" which revealed that 12.6% experienced discrimination infrequently whilst 5.9% experienced discrimination frequently.

5. Conclusion

The study established that many respondents believed that most healthcare facilities are not physically accessible due to the absence of ramps and elevators. Respondents are discriminated against and stigmatized both in hospitals and on public transport. It was also found that many public means of transport are not accessible to children with CP. Respondents believed that the National Health Policy is ineffective and the NHIS does not cover a wide range of services for children with CP. Moreover, the study also pointed out that the majority of the respondents seek medical care for their children with CP however others also seek spiritual healing for their children with CP.

Author details

Nathaniel Larbi Andah
Social and Behavioral Science Department, School of Public Health - University of Ghana, Greater Accra, Ghana

*Address all correspondence to: nathdarko@gmail.com

References

[1] United Nations. United Nations Web Services Section, Department of Public Information. Convention on the Rights for Persons with Disabilities: Some facts about persons with disabilities; 2006. Available from: http://www.un.org/disabilities/convention/facts.shtml on 9th October 2019

[2] World Health Organization World report on disability: Main report (Malta ed. Vol. 1 of 2): World Health Organization and the World Bank; 2015

[3] Janzek-hawlat S. Impact of waiting times in health care. June 2015. DOI: 10.13140/RG.2.1.4164.6240

[4] UN General Assembly. Convention on the rights of persons with disabilities: Resolution/adopted by the General Assembly, 24 January 2007, A/RES/61/106, Available from: https://www.refworld.org/docid/45f973632.html [Accessed 15 June 2021]

[5] Singogo C, Mweshi M, Rhoda A. Challenges experienced by mothers caring for children with cerebral palsy in Zambia. South African Journal of Physiotherapy. 2015;**71**(1):1-6. DOI: 10.4102/sajp.v71i1.274

[6] Opoku MP, Alupo BA, Gyamfi N, Mprah W. The family and disability in Ghana: Highlighting gaps in achieving social inclusion. (March). 2018. DOI: 10.5463/dcid.v28i4.666

[7] Tudzi EP, Bugri JT, Danso AK. Human rights of students with disabilities in ghana: Accessibility of the university built environment human rights of students with disabilities in Ghana: Accessibility of the University Built Environment. 8131(September). 2017. DOI: 10.1080/18918131.2017.1348678

[8] World Health Organization. International Classification of Functioning, Disability and Health (ICF). Geneva: World Health Organization; 2011a

[9] World Health Organization. World report on disability: Main report. Malta ed. Vol. 1 of 2. World Health Organization and the World Bank; 2011b

[10] Smide B, Aarts C. Family perceptions in caring for children and adolescents with mental disabilities: A qualitative study from Tanzania. Journal of Health Research. 2010;**12**(2)129-137

[11] Cristina Atendido MM, Candidate L. Discrimination in health care against persons with disabilities the ADA on health. 12181(7), 12182. 2013. Available from: http://www.ada.gov/medcare_mobility_ta/medcare_ta.htm

[12] Google map. Health districts in greater Accra list of hospitals in Ghana - Wikipedia. 2019

[13] Levesque J-F, Harris MF, Russell G. Patient-centred access to health care: Conceptualising access at the interface of health systems and populations. International Journal for Equity in Health. 2013;**12**(1):1-9

[14] Khatri RB, Karkee R. Social determinants of health affecting utilization of routine maternity services in Nepal: A narrative review of the evidence. Reproductive Health Matters. 2018a;**26**(54):32-46. DOI: 10.1080/09688080.2018.1535686

[15] Vartan CK, Montuschi E. National health policy. British Medical Journal. 2020;**2**(4312):279. DOI: 10.1136/bmj.2.4312.279

[16] Akande AA, Akande TM. Awareness and attitude of medical practitioners in Ilorin towards the National Health Insurance Scheme. Sahel Medical Journal. 2003;**6**(1):14-16

[17] Dixon J, Tenkorang EY, Luginaah I. Ghana's National health insurance scheme: A national-level investigation of members' perceptions of service provision. BMC International Health and Human Rights. 2013;**13**(1):1-10. DOI: 10.1186/1472-698X-13-35

[18] Gopalan SS, Durairaj V. Addressing women's non-maternal healthcare financing in developing countries: What can we learn from the experiences of rural Indian women? PLoS One. 2012;**7**:8

[19] Bruce E, Narh-Bana S, Agyepong I. Community satisfaction, equity in coverage, and implications for sustainability of the dangme west health insurance scheme. Project No. 2001/GD/08. Technical Report Series No. 9. Accra: Ghanaian Dutch Collaboration for Health Research and Development. 2008

[20] Dalinjong PA, Laar AS. The national health insurance scheme: Perceptions and experiences of health care providers and clients in two districts of Ghana. Health Economics Review. 2012;**2**:13. DOI: 10.1186/2191-1991-2-13

[21] Boz C, Sur H, Soyuk S. The affecting factors of healthcare services demand in terms of health services use: A field application. International Journal of Health and Life Sciences. 2016;**1**(2):33-41

[22] Matt SB. Perceptions of disability among caregivers of children with disabilities in Nicaragua: Implications for future opportunities and health care access. International Journal of Medical and Public Health. 2014:1-17

[23] Centers for Disease Control and Prevention. Causes and risk factors of cerebral palsy. 2019. Retrieved from: https://www.cdc.gov/ncbddd/cp/causes.html

[24] Cerebral Palsy Alliance. Signs and symptoms of cerebral palsy. 2018. Retrieved from: https://cerebralpalsy.org.au/our-research/about-cerebral-palsy/what-is-cerebralpalsy/signs-and-symptoms-of-cp/

[25] Cerebral Palsy Guide. Treatment for cerebral palsy. 2020. Retrieved from: https://www.cerebralpalsyguide.com/cerebral-palsy/

[26] Physioplus. Parents of children with cerebral palsy; raising a child with cerebral palsy. 2020. Retrieved from: https://www.physiopedia.com/Parents_of_Children_with_Cerebral_Palsy

[27] Butchner P. Society's attitude towards persons with disabilities. 2020. Retrieved from: https://paul-burtner.dental.ufl.edu/oral-health-care-for-persons-with-disabilities/societysattitude-toward-people-with-disabilities/

[28] Duran S, Ergün S. The stigma perceived by parents of intellectual disability children: An interpretative phenomenological analysis study Yorumlayıcı bir fenomenolojik analiz çalışması. 2018. DOI: 10.5455/apd.282536

[29] DeVoe JE, Tillotson CJ, Wallace LS. Insurance coverage gaps among US children with insured parents: Are middle-income children more likely to have longer gaps? Maternal and Child Health Journal. 2011;**15**(3):342-351

[30] Review AS, Africaine R. Employment status, medical support, and income as significant factors in access to essential. Medicine. 2017;**21**(1):154-175

[31] Bulamu Healthcare. The State of Healthcare in Uganda. 2019. Retrieved from: https://bulamuhealthcare.org/healthcare-in-uganda/

[32] Balcı NÇ. We are IntechOpen, the world's leading publisher of Open Access books Built by scientists, for scientists' TOP 1%. 2016

[33] Awoyemi TT, Obayelu OA, Opaluwa HI. Effect of distance on utilization of health care services in Rural Kogi State, Nigeria. Journal of Human Ecology. 2011;**35**(1):1-9. DOI: 10.1080/09709274.2011.11906385

[34] Nesbitt RC, Lohela TJ, Soremekun S, Vesel L, Manu A, Okyere E, et al. The influence of distance and quality of care on a place of delivery in rural Ghana. Scientific Reports. 2016;**6**(June):1-8. DOI: 10.1038/srep30291

[35] World Health Organization. The need to scale up a rehabilitation. Rehabilitation. 2017;**2**(2):1-9. Available from: https://www.who.int/disabilities/care/ NeedToScaleUpRehab.pdf%0Ahttp:// www.who.int/disabilities/care/Need-to-scale-up-rehab-July2018.pdf?ua=1

[36] Jamshidi S, Parker JS, Hashemi S. The effects of environmental factors on the patient outcomes in hospital environments: A review of the literature. Frontiers of Architectural Research. 2020;**9**(2):249-263. DOI: 10.1016/j.foar.2019.10.001

[37] Douglas CH, Douglas MR. Patient-friendly hospital environments: Exploring the patients' perspective. Health Expectations. 2004;**7**(1):61-73. DOI: 10.1046/j.1369-6513.2003.00251.x

[38] Rogers SE, Thrasher AD, Miao Y, Boscardin WJ, Smith AK. Discrimination in healthcare settings is associated with disability in older adults: Health and retirement study, 2008-2012. Journal of General Internal Medicine. 2015;**30**(10):1413-1420. DOI: 10.1007/s11606-015-3233-6

Chapter 7

The Japan Obstetric Compensation System for Cerebral Palsy: Novel System to Improve Quality and Safety in Perinatal Care and Mitigate Conflict

Shin Ushiro

Abstract

The Japan Obstetric Compensation System for Cerebral Palsy was launched in 2009 in response to a shortage of obstetricians and a surge in disputes. The system is characterized by the provision of no-fault compensation, investigation, and prevention. We have certified more than 3000 cerebral palsy cases for compensation and have delivered investigative reports, prevention reports, and educative media for professionals and expectant mothers. We have also produced recapitulation of individual investigative report to be uploaded on the webpage of the system to enhance transparency. The disclosure is reviewed to be consistent with lately revised Personal Information Protection Law in 2020. In order to expand the system by revising eligibility criteria, the system was and will be reviewed in 2015 and 2022. The new criteria that were crafted in ad-hoc committee in 2019–2020 will be applied in 2022 and later. As such, the system has been a significant part of perinatal care delivery system in Japan.

Keywords: cerebral palsy, the Japan Obstetric Compensation System for Cerebral Palsy, Japan Council for Quality Healthcare, no-fault compensation

1. Introduction

The Japan Obstetric Compensation System for Cerebral Palsy [1–4] was launched in 2009 by the Japan Council for Quality Health Care (JQ) as operating organization, with the background of a shortage of obstetricians in Japan and a surge in disputes particularly caused by occurrence of cerebral palsy (CP). More than 10 years have passed since the system commenced, and it has given rise to enormous achievements such as early resolution of disputes displayed in the rapid decrease in the number of lawsuit statistics and quality improvement of perinatal care. It is of note that the system was designed in an introductory committee in the presence of range of stakeholders such as professional organizations, academic organizations, insurance firm, lawyers, and patient representatives. They have been involved in implementing the

IntechOpen

system that was helpful in obtaining confidence in the system. Here, in this article, current status of the system and challenges ahead are described.

2. Background to the launch the system

2.1 Perinatal care and conflict

Among the disputes, those related to cerebral palsy were said to be a heavy burden for obstetricians because the cause of cerebral palsy was often unknown. In discussions with perinatal care professionals in Japan and abroad, it has been said that cerebral palsy is one of the causes of disputes, including court cases, and of obstetricians leaving their jobs, not only in high-income countries but also in middle-low-income countries (LMICs). In cases where a child is born in a distressed status despite normal course of pregnancy and delivery, or where the child's neurological deficits become apparent to develop profound cerebral palsy in spite of little or no findings on hypoxic condition during delivery, the family's sentiment may become complicated due to uncertainty on the cause of cerebral palsy and a dispute may arise. Therefore, obstetricians had been discussing for many years the establishment of a compensation system that runs on no-fault basis in anticipation for mitigating the conflict.

2.2 Deliberation on establishing no-fault compensation system

Discussions on the establishment of a no-fault compensation system have been held by the Japan Medical Association (JMA) since the 1960s. In the report entitled "Report on the Legal Response to Medical Accidents and Its Basic Theory" published in 1972, the following recommendations were set forth [5].

i. In the event of a medical accident, if the physician's practices are deemed to be negligent through a rigorous examination, he or she will be immediately held responsible for compensation.

ii. Compensation should be established on a national scale to provide relief for serious damage inevitably caused by physicians whose practices are not negligent.

iii. The establishment of a dispute resolution procedure as a national system separate from the current court system.

The JMA physician liability insurance system was established in 1973 in response to (i), but the other two items were not materialized for decades that followed. With decades passing by, the shortage of physicians in obstetrics and gynecology and the declining birthrate became social problems. In January 2006, the JMA made a proposition in its report entitled "Aiming at the establishment of a disability compensation system for medical care" stating "Ideally, it is desirable to implement a no-fault compensation system for entire medical specialties" and "however, neurological sequelae related to childbirth (so-called cerebral palsy) is prioritized for no-fault compensation." In August of the same year, they presented the details on the novel system [6]. Furthermore, in November of the year, "A Framework for a No-Fault Compensation System in Obstetrics" (Study Group on Medical Dispute Resolution, Social Security

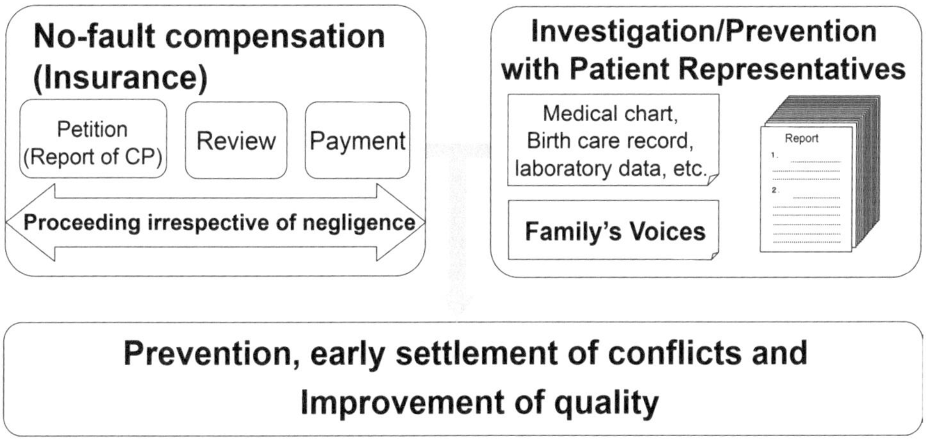

Figure 1.
No-fault compensation/investigation/prevention system for cerebral palsy, 2009.

System Study Group, Political Research Committee of the Liberal Democratic Party (LDP)) was published that was followed by growing anticipation to launch the system. It depicted that the novel system is equipped with two pillars such as compensation on no-fault basis and investigation and prevention. At the same time, relevant organizations and groups expressed their concern and requested that the JQ should be an operator of the system. Accordingly, the Preparatory Office for the novel system was installed in the JQ in February 2007 that served as secretariat for the Introductory Committee for the novel system. In March 2008, the Board of Directors of the JQ formally decided to be the operating organization. All in this way, the system has been in operation since January 2009 (**Figure 1**).

2.3 Registration of childbirth facility

The system was launched and being hailed by professional societies such as the Japan Association of Obstetricians and Gynecologists (JAOG) and Japanese Midwife Association (JMA). They, therefore, helped the JQ to involve childbirth facilities across Japan for registration in the system. Although there is no legislation that mandates them participate in the system, the JQ successfully observed extremely high registration rate in the system as high as 99.9% achieved in close cooperation with the societies and relevant stakeholders [7] (**Table 1**).

Type of facility	No. childbirth facilities	No. participating facilities	% Participation
Hospital	1173	1173	100.0
Clinic	1557	1555	99.9
Birth center	445	445	100.0
Total	3175	3173	99.9*

**Institutions not registered: 2 clinics.*

Table 1.
Registration rate by type of facility. As of November 30, 2021.

2.4 Review and compensation

The scope of those eligible for compensation must meet the general criteria, which consists of birth weight and weeks of pregnancy, or the individual criteria when the weeks of pregnancy are less than the general criteria : 28 weeks or more of pregnancy, case-by-case criteria: umbilical artery blood pH less than 7.1, meeting one of the prescribed patterns in the fetal heart rate labor diagram (CTG) that indicate hypoxia in the fetus, etc., meets severity criteria: degree equivalent to level 1 or 2 of the physical disability grade defined in the Welfare for the Disabled Act, and does not meet the exclusion criteria such as cerebral palsy obviously caused by congenital factors or factors taking place in neonatal period and later [8]. Even if congenital factors (brain malformation, genetic abnormality, chromosomal abnormality, etc.) exist, patients are not necessarily excluded because the factors may not be the obvious cause of profound CP. Decision for approval is made based on medical examination as to what caused profound CP that applicant suffers. The general criteria and case-by-case criteria were revised in reference to aggregated data and scientific progress on cerebral palsy. The latest criteria that applied to cerebral palsy who were born in 2022 or later does not include case-by-case criteria due to expansion of general criteria so that more cerebral palsy would be covered (**Table 2**). The revision of the criteria is described later.

As of June 2021, 3374 cases have been approved for compensation, and payment for the cases have been swiftly made or in progress. The annual number of persons eligible for compensation to such criteria as 2009 and 2015 criteria that have been confirmed so far is 419 in 2009, 382 in 2010, 355 in 2011, 362 in 2012, 351 in 2013, 326 in 2014, and 376 in 2015. For children born in later years, the application is still allowed until they are 5 years old (**Table 3**). It should be noted that the number of approved patients rose to a certain extent in 2015 because new criteria that could cover more cerebral palsy were applied. In addition, applicants of uncompensated cases may apply to the Appeal Committee if they are not convinced on the results of the review.

A uniform compensation of 30 million yen is paid for each case once approved by the Review Committee. There are two different ways applied to the payment such as lumpsum payment and annual installment that continue 20 times (**Figure 2**). If child-birth facility is liable for the development of cerebral palsy, the compensation and the damage payment are adjusted to eliminate duplicative payments. In other words, the child and the family cannot receive both the compensation and the damage payment in the system [9].

3. Investigation

3.1 Production of investigative report

The purpose of the investigation is (i) to analyze the case from a medical point of view based on record and data on the cerebral palsy to learn knowledge for prevention and (ii) prevent conflict between childbirth facility and patient/family and bring it to early settlement by sharing investigative report for mutual understanding on the childbirth event. Unlike court system, this is a process of analysis genuinely from medical and midwifery point of view [10].

	2009–2014	2015–2021	2022–
General criteria	33rd week or later and 2000 g or over	32nd week or later and 1400 g or over	28th week or later
Case-by-Case	"28th week or later" AND "A) OR B)" (A) Umbilical cord arterial blood pH; less than 7.1 (B) Specific deceleration patterns* on CTG * Any patterns of "a" AND "any of b-d" a. Loss of variability of the baseline b. Late decelerations observed at 50% or over of uterine contractions c. Variable decelerations observed at 50% or over of uterine contractions d. Severe bradycardia with reduced variability of the baseline	"28th week or later" AND "A) OR B)" (A) Umbilical cord arterial blood pH; less than 7.1 (B) Specific deceleration patterns* on CTG * Any patterns of a-h" a. Abrupt and persistent bradycardia b. Late decelerations observed at 50% or over of uterine contractions c. Variable decelerations observed at 50% or over of uterine contractions d. Loss of variability of the baseline e. Severe deceleration with loss of variability of the baseline f. Sinusoidal pattern g. Apgar score at 3 or less at 1 min after birth h. Arterial blood gas pH less than 7.0 within 1 hour after birth	None
Exclusion	a. Congenital causes Bilateral diffuse cerebral malformation, chromosomal disorders, genetic disorders, congenital metabolic disorders or other congenital abnormalities b. Neonatal causes Encephalitis, brain injuries etc. that obviously take place after birth	a. Congenital causes Bilateral diffuse cerebral malformation, chromosomal disorders, genetic disorders, congenital metabolic disorders or other congenital abnormalities b. Neonatal causes Encephalitis, brain injuries etc. that obviously take place after birth	a. Congenital causes Bilateral diffuse cerebral malformation, chromosomal disorders, genetic disorders, congenital metabolic disorders or other congenital abnormalities b. Neonatal causes Encephalitis, brain injuries etc. that obviously take place after birth
Impairment degree	1st-2nd degree i.g. wheelchair defined in the Act on Social Care for the Disabled	1st-2nd degree i.g. wheelchair defined in the Act on Social Care for the Disabled	1st-2nd degree i.g. wheelchair defined in the Act on Social Care for the Disabled

Table 2.
Eligibility criteria: criteria of 2009, 2015 and 2022.

The Investigation Committee holds seven subcommittees to compile a draft report (**Figure 3**). One committee is composed of 14 members: nine obstetricians including the chairperson, two pediatricians, one midwife, and two lawyers. The role of the medical members is to analyze the case from medical viewpoint, while the lawyers provide views so that the report will be easy for patient/family to understand. A working manual was crafted to ensure that the reports are compiled in standardized fashion. The draft report compiled therein is reviewed in the Investigative Committee for approval. At the same time, a "summarized edition" of the investigative report is issued with personal identifiers deleted and held available on the system's website for prevention and improvement of perinatal care.

Birth year	No. case reviewed	Eligible	Not-Eligible				Petition
		Eligible	Not Eligible	Preliminary to review	Total	Review in progress	
2009	561	419	142	0	142	0	Expired
2010	523	382	141	0	141	0	Expired
2011	502	355	147	0	147	0	Expired
2012	517	361	155	0	155	0	Expired
2013	476	351	125	0	125	0	Expired
2014	469	326	143	0	143	0	Expired
2015	475	376	99	0	99	0	Expired
2016–2019	933	803	81	41	122	8	Valid
Total	4456	3374	1033	41	1,074	11	

Table 3.
Statistics of eligible case by birth year.

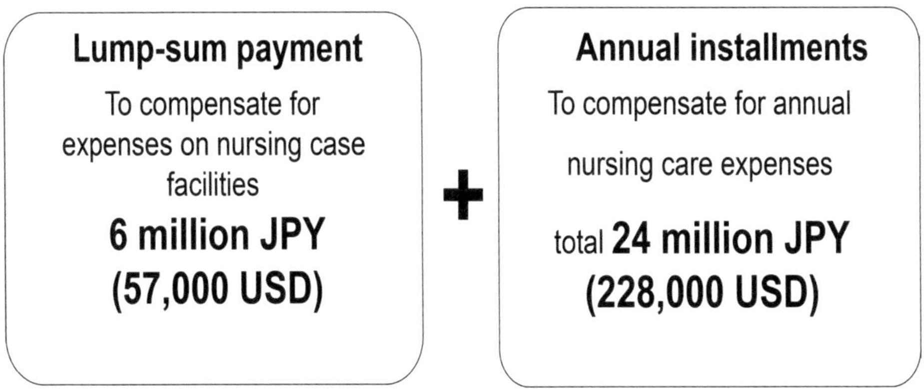

Figure 2.
Sum of compensation payment (30 million JPY = 342,000 USD).

3.2 The relationship between the disclosure of the "Synthesized edition" of the investigative report and the latest revision of the Personal Information Protection Law and relevant administrative guidelines

The "Synthesized edition" of the investigative report has been published and posted on the website as one of the products of the system [11]. They have been referred by parents, patient groups, and medical professionals for various purposes such as confirming transparency and improving quality of perinatal care through scientific research. The revised Act on the Protection of Personal Information was enacted and promulgated in 2015 and fully enforced on May 30, 2017, which unprecedentedly forced the "Donor rule" applicable when we consider if the data we disclose on the web is "Personal information." "Personal information" shall be provided to third parties through the prior consent of an individual to which the data belong with some exceptions such as the data provision for promoting public health. The "Donor rule" states that the data is defined as "Personal information" when the

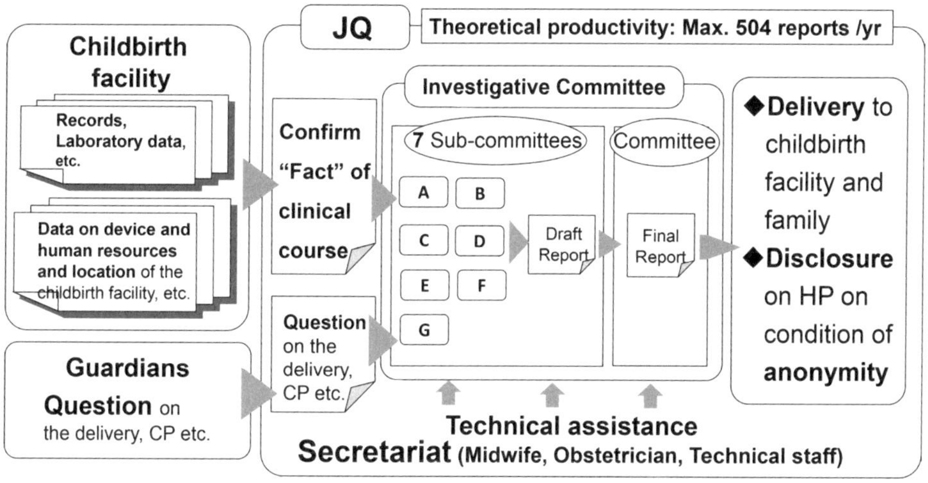

Figure 3.
Production of standardized investigative report.

donor of the data, i.e., the JQ can identify an individual from whom the data derive even if recipient of the data, i.e., the general public does not know whose data it is. Accordingly, the "Synthesized edition" that had been available on the website turned out to be "Personal information" that could be transferred to third parties principally through prior consent procedure. Therefore, the "Synthesized edition" posted on the website, for which consent of family and childbirth facility for the disclosure had not been obtained, had to be temporarily withdrawn from the website, and the Steering Committee took deeper dive into the issue from a broad perspectives such as purpose and impact of the disclosure and procedures required for the disclosure in consistent with the revised Personal Information Protection Act [12].

In January 2019, the JQ consulted with legal experts and the government officials again on this issue. In light of their comments and guidance, the JQ decided to make efforts in obtaining the consent of the guardians, the childbirth institutions, and the relevant medical institutions on all the "Synthesized editions" in response to the public concern on the system and the changing public view with regard to the handling of personal information, although the JQ believed that it fell under the exceptions for obtaining prior consent to the provision of personal information to third parties in the revised Personal Information Protection Act (**Table 4**). Later, when the JQ's policy on disclosure of the "Synthesized edition" was proposed at the 40th Steering Committee meeting held in January 2019, comments such as "all synthesized editions should be disclosed on the web as they were" and "The JQ should clarify the reasons for no-consent by guardians and/or childbirth facilities in detail" were raised from many of committee members.

Article 23 A business operator handling personal information shall not provide personal data to a third party without obtaining the prior consent of the individual, except in the following cases (i)-(ii) Omitted. (iii) When it is particularly necessary for the improvement of public health or the promotion of the sound growth of children, and it is difficult to obtain the consent of the person concerned.

Table 4.
Article 23, paragraph 1, item 3 of the Personal Information Protection Act.

In February 2019, the JQ conducted a questionnaire survey targeting guardians and childbirth facilities to get hold of the reasons why they answered "agree" or "disagree" on the disclosure of the "Synthesized edition." At the 41st Steering Committee meeting held in August 2019, the JQ reviewed the aim and value of this system to consider if we should disclose all the "Synthesized edition" that achieves public good such as quality improvement in perinatal care as only about 3/4 of the "Synthesized edition" is agreed on the disclosure [13]. The JQ concluded at that time that it continued its efforts to improve the rate of consent on disclosure and consulted with the relevant ministries and the government to explore measures to disclose more "Synthesized editions" on the web.

In December 2019, the Personal Information Protection Committee in the government published the "Outline of the Amendment of the System for the So-called Triennial Review of the Personal Information Protection Act" (**Table 5**), and in January 2020, the Ministry of Health, Labor and Welfare (MHLW) presented a new commentary (**Table 6**). At the 42nd Steering Committee held in February 2020 and the 43rd Steering Committee meeting held on July 3, this issue was discussed to eventually compile an audacious policy on releasing all the "Synthesized editions" on the web. In the meantime, at the 94th meeting of the Investigation Committee

3. Clarification of the exception defined in the law pertaining to the handling of personal information for the purpose of public interest With the rapid progress of information and communication technology, it has become possible to collect and analyze big data such as customer information. In this context, Japan is aiming to realize Society 5.0, which is a new society in which advanced technologies such as big data analysis are incorporated into all industries and social life to achieve both economic development and solutions to social issues. As social issues become more diverse, it is desirable to support an environment in which businesses can make use of data in order to efficiently and effectively solve these issues. With regard to this point, the current Personal Information Protection Act has exceptions to the limitation of the purpose of use and provision to third parties, such as "when it is necessary for the protection of the life, body, or property of an individual and it is difficult to obtain the consent of the individual" and "when it is particularly necessary for the improvement of public health or the promotion of the sound growth of children and it is difficult to obtain the consent of the individual." The use of personal information for public benefit is also considered acceptable in certain cases. However, since there is a tendency that these exceptions have been strictly applied so far, it is necessary to provide specific examples in guidelines and Q&As according to the expected needs. Therefore, we will promote the utilization of personal information that benefits the entire nation, such as the resolution of social issues, by providing specific examples in the guidelines and Q&As according to the expected needs. For example, a case in which a medical institution or a pharmaceutical manufacturer uses the information for the purpose of contributing to the development of medical research in order to realize healthcare services, drugs, and medical devices of high quality in terms of safety and effectiveness.

Table 5.
The Personal Information Protection Law, dubbed as Triennial Review, Outline of System Revisions (December 13, 2019) (excerpt).

In December 2019, the Personal Information Protection Committee released the "Personal Information Protection Act: dubbed as Triennial Review: Outline of Revisions," which also states that "the handling of personal information in the private sector is a matter for each business operator to decide. Therefore, it would be desirable for the JQ to consider the policy again, taking into account the balance between the promotion of public health and the protection of personal information. In addition, the MHLW has no objection if it is widely accepted by the society to disclose the summarized edition of all investigative reports as they were."

Table 6.
Commentary issued to the JQ by the Ministry of Health, Labor and Welfare.

held on June 10, the following comments to support the full disclosure were proposed: "In the Investigative Report, the causes of cerebral palsy are analyzed in detail and carefully for each case. So, they are worthwhile to disclose, and "All the "Synthesized editions" need to be disclosed on the web as they were. Accordingly, it was unanimously agreed that the "Synthesized edition" is published for all the Investigation Reports. From the viewpoint of improving public health, the publication of the "Synthesized edition" falls under the exceptions of Article 23, Paragraph 1, Item 3 of the Personal Information Protection Act as described above (**Table 4**). In addition, in order to prevent the recurrence of CPs, which is the purpose of the system, and to widely commit to quality improvement in perinatal care, the JQ believed that it was incredibly important to disclose all "Synthesized edition" on the web after a year-long argument over the disclosure under the revised Personal Information Protection Act. As there were some opinions that a certain level of agreement has been formed between the JQ and the family and childbirth facility who had disagreed on the disclosure, the JQ needed to make efforts to carefully convince families and childbirth facilities to agree on the new policy on disclosure. After all those discussions, the new disclosure policy was agreed in the Steering Committee [14].

4. Prevention of cerebral palsy

4.1 Publication of annual prevention reports, educational materials on fetal heart rate monitoring, and leaflets for professionals and expectant mothers

The investigative reports are collectively analyzed in order to prevent recurrence and to improve quality in perinatal care [15]. Here, we applied the knowledge and procedure devised through the medical adverse event reporting and learning system that the JQ had run for more than a decade to produce materials for effective prevention of CP through collective analysis. Specifically, the JQ conducted a quantitative and epidemiological analysis of aggregated cases to produce report for prevention on annual basis based on such data as status of pregnancy, clinical courses of pregnancy, delivery and neonatal condition, and the local context of healthcare delivery system [16]. The JQ also produced educational materials such as fetal heart rate monitoring textbook of profound CPs and leaflets for medical professionals and pregnant women [17].

4.2 Scientific achievements of the Prevention Working Group

Under the Prevention Committee, a working group for prevention, which consists of obstetricians nominated by the Japan Society of Obstetrics and Gynecology (JSOG) and the Japan Association of Obstetricians and Gynecologists (JAOG), as well as academic experts such as epidemiologists, was established in May 2014 that has carried out data analysis of the aggregated Investigative Reports. With the data, comparative study between the data of CPs that were subject to compensation in this system and that of the "Japan Society of Obstetrics and Gynecology Perinatal Registration Database" was conducted. In addition, an analysis of intrauterine infections and fetal heart rate patterns in children with CP was conducted in response to the requests mentioned in the Prevention Report to the relevant academic societies and organizations. The analyses have been

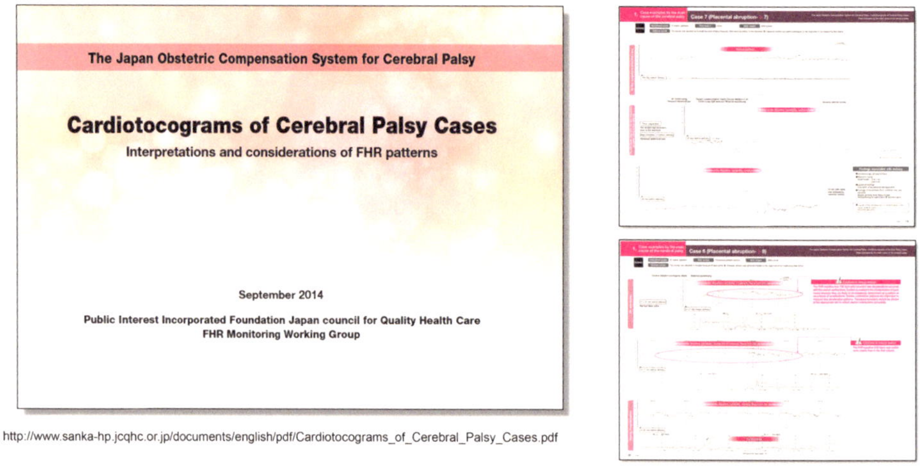

Figure 4.
Educative book on CTG pattern of CPs.

implemented in the working group from such multifaceted viewpoints as obstetrics and public health.

As the system requests that childbirth facility submit application with relevant documents such as medical chart, cardiotocogram (CTG) recording and so on, the system happened to provided experts an opportunity to scientifically look into CTG data through collective analysis. It is normally difficult in Japan to obtain CTG data of profound cerebral palsy as it suddenly happens at any childbirth facility across the country. Taking advantage of the considerable number of CTG recordings, the experts published an educational book on CTG interpretation, which is available on the website of the system (**Figure 4**) [18].

4.3 Impact on lawsuit statistics

The purpose of the system is to prevent disputes and to improve quality in perinatal care through no-fault compensation, investigation/prevention. The lawsuit statistics of obstetrics and gynecology as a breakdown of "the number of completed lawsuit of entire medical specialty" published by the Committee on Medical Lawsuit of the Supreme Court of Japan shows a remarkable decreasing trend (**Figure 5**). The "Report on the Verification of the Speeding Up of Trials" published in July 2013 by the Supreme Court of Japan stated that: [19]

> *"It is noteworthy that the Japan Obstetric Compensation System for Cerebral Palsy has brought investigative system by a third party and system of equally imposing financial burden for monetary compensation in Japanese society sharing the idea that perinatal care inherently holds potential risk.*
>
> *It is concerned whether the system expands to cover other medical specialties.*
>
> *The system having approved significant number of CP cases supposedly has affected to a certain extent statistics of lawsuit cases of medicine."*

As such, the system was hailed not only by medical society but by legal circle in Japan. As described in the report, medical professionals anticipated to expand

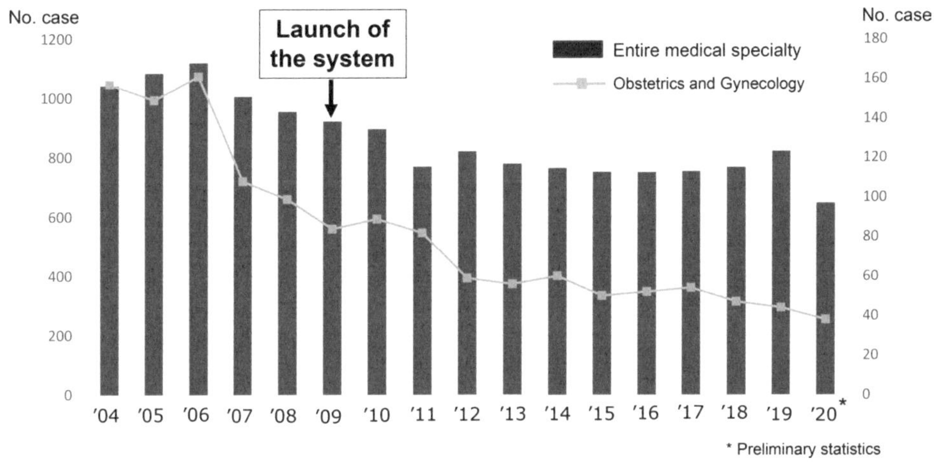

Figure 5.
Lawsuit statistics 2004–2020.

the system or launch a similar system to cover more clinical specialties. However, there has never been emergence of desire in medical society comparable to the one observed in late 2000s that led to the launch of the system for cerebral palsy. Therefore, the expansion is still under discussion in academic society such as the Japan Surgical Society.

5. Review and overhaul of the system: 2015 and 2022

5.1 Timetable for review and overhaul agreed at the inception of the system

The Japan Obstetric Compensation System for Cerebral Palsy was launched in expedited manner in the wake of deteriorating perinatal care delivery system with challenges difficult to address at the time of the inception. Therefore, the report of the Introductory Committee stated that "the system will be verified in five years at the latest, and necessary revisions will be made to the scope of eligible patients, the amount of monetary compensation, price of insurance premium, and the governing structure of the system as appropriate. As such, periodical review and overhaul has been systematically embedded in the system" [20–24].

5.2 2015 Overhaul

Accordingly, the Steering Committee of the system began deliberation over the review of the system in February 2012. The committee conducted fact-finding research including the collection and analysis of population-based data on the incidence of cerebral palsy, which is necessary for estimating the number of eligible patient and is crucial for re-designing the system. The results were reported to the Steering Committee in July 2013, and the committee and the Medical Insurance Subcommittee of the Social Security Council of the MHLW reviewed to revamp the system in terms of the scope of eligibility, the amount of monetary compensation, the price of insurance premium, and the way to spend surplus that had aggregated since the launch of the system. The review concluded that the system expanded the scope of eligibility with the same amount of monetary compensation to be applied in January 2015 and later. As to how to spend growing surplus, the Medical Insurance Subcommittee agreed that the insurance premium was reduced to the price that work with the surplus to sustainably ensure budget for compensation. It was planned that the surplus was spent for the next 10 years by 2024 to consume it.

5.3 2022 Overhaul

With the system being run carrying out the revised eligibility criteria, the Steering Committee meeting held on July 20, 2018, found that such issues had arisen as "more than 50% of the patients on case-by-case review were not covered by the system", "a sense of unfairness is spreading because some patients were covered and others were not despite of suffering commonly from CP with similar clinical course," and "the revised criteria has already been inconsistent with the latest knowledge from scientific viewpoint." Therefore, it was concluded that the system needed to be revised as soon as possible. In July of the same year, the Steering Committee submitted a request to the MHLW that the committee commenced the review of the system to overhaul because the MHLW is authorized to fix the price of childbirth lumpsum payment under the government regulation that substantially gives rise to financial source of compensation. Later in the year, the MHLW responded to the JQ claiming that the JQ listens to the voices of relevant parties such as healthcare-related entities, patient groups, and insurers, proposes the blueprint to reform the system, and reports the conclusion to the MHLW so that the MHLW would take necessary action for the reform.

With those dialogs between the JQ and the MHLW, the first round of the Committee on the Review of the Japan Obstetric Compensation System for Cerebral Palsy was held on September 2020. At the meeting, the items to be examined and reviewed were presented to the committee members such as "Efficiency in running the system," "Latest estimates of the number of eligible patients," "Price of insurance premium," "Eligibility criteria for compensation," "Financial resource for compensation," and "Price of compensation." The JQ engaged in Q&A session in the committee in exploring the expansion of the system, which was in line with the views of the most committee members who engaged in perinatal care. In addition to the agreement with members with healthcare background, it was necessary to make efforts to reach a unanimous agreement of the stakeholders including public health insurers involved in the meeting. Therefore, the JQ requested committee members and all those involved in perinatal care across the country for attention and support for the direction, i.e., expansion of the system that JQ proposed in response to the difficult reality in perinatal care delivery system.

The Committee compiled a report on the blueprint of the revision to submit to the MHLW subcommittee on healthcare insurance that works under the MHLW Social Security Panel. The subcommittee includes members such as healthcare insurers, academic experts, and representatives of healthcare professionals, industries, and labor unions. It endorsed the report in December 2020 that led to the launch of the revised system in January 2022 (**Table 2**).

5.4 Future implication of the no-fault compensation system

The Japan Obstetrics Compensation System for Cerebral Palsy, which was launched in 2009, celebrated its tenth anniversary in 2019. During this period, the system has made enormous achievements such as delivery of no-fault compensation for profound CPs, provision of investigative report to share both with families and childbirth facilities, prevention activities through collective analysis of aggregated investigative reports, and sharing plenty of scientific data on CPs gained through the system on a national scale. The system was reviewed 5 years after it was launched on a planned timetable produced initially. The review concluded that the system was run appropriately in line with the original objectives, such as provision of monetary compensation on no-fault basis, early resolution of disputes, and quality improvement of perinatal care through investigation and prevention. Then, the revised system was partly initiated in January 2014 on such details as procedure of investigation and adjustment of monetary compensation and damage payment, and in January 2015 on the rest of the details such as scope of eligibility to cover more CPs and other issues relevant to insurance. The JQ completed another review of the system to explore further expansion to cover more cerebral palsy cases in January 2022 and later. As seen above, the JQ believes that it is vital to improve the system in continued fashion through periodical review in cooperation with stakeholders.

Author details

Shin Ushiro[1,2]

1 Japan Council for Quality Health Care (JQ), Japan

2 Division of Patient Safety, Kyushu University Hospital, Japan

*Address all correspondence to: ushiro.shin.161@m.kyushu-u.ac.jp

References

[1] Website of the Japan Obstetric Compensation for Cerebral Palsy (Top Page). Available from: http://www.sanka-hp.jcqhc.or.jp/ [Accessed: June 01, 2022, in Japanese]

[2] Website of the Japan Obstetric Compensation for Cerebral Palsy (Leaflet of the Japan Obstetric Compensation System for Cerebral Palsy (for Guardians)). Available from: http://www.sanka-hp.jcqhc.or.jp/documents/english/pdf/seidoannnaitirashi_english_202106.pdf [Accessed: June 01, 2022, in English]

[3] Website of the Japan Obstetric Compensation for Cerebral Palsy (Brochure on the Japan Obstetric Compensation System for Cerebral Palsy – Achievements through 10-years. Available from: http://www.sanka-hp.jcqhc.or.jp/documents/english/pdf/looking_back_over10years_after_system_was_launched201906.pdf [Accessed: June 01, 2022, in English]

[4] Ushiro S et al. Japan Obstetric Compensation for Cerebral Palsy: Strategic system fof data aggregation, investigation, amelioration and no-fault compensation. Journal of Obstetrics and Gynaecology Research. 2019;**45**(3):493-513

[5] Committee on Legal Affair, Japan Medical Association. A report on "Legal proceedings for medical accidents and the relevant theory". Journal of Japan MEdical Association. 1972;**68**:183-203

[6] Study Group on the Compensation for the Disability Associated Medicine. Report on "Toward the Compensation to a Case that Happens in Association with Medical Management and Procedure" by the Japan Medical Association. Material of the 1st meeting of the Planning Committee of the Japan Obstetric Compensation System for Cerebral Palsy (JOCSCP), Japan Council for Quality Health Care; 2008. pp. 1-10. Available from: http://www.sanka-hp.jcqhc.or.jp/documents/committee/pdf/obstetrics_3.pdf [Accessed: June 01, 2022, in Japanese]

[7] Website of the Japan Obstetric Compensation for Cerebral Palsy (Registration Data of Medical Institutions). Available from: http://www.sanka-hp.jcqhc.or.jp/search/kanyujokyo.php [Accessed: June 01, 2022, in Japanese]

[8] Website of the Japan Obstetric Compensation for Cerebral Palsy (Eligibility Criteria). Available from: http://www.sanka-hp.jcqhc.or.jp/application/sphere.html [Accessed: June 01, 2022, in Japanese]

[9] Website of the Japan Obstetric Compensation for Cerebral Palsy (Procedure for Receiving Compensation Payment). Available from: http://www.sanka-hp.jcqhc.or.jp/outline/compensation.html [Accessed: June 01, 2022, in Japanese]

[10] Website of the Japan Obstetric Compensation for Cerebral Palsy (Investigation). Available from: http://www.sanka-hp.jcqhc.or.jp/outline/function.html [Accessed: June 01, 2022, in Japanese]

[11] Website of the Japan Obstetric Compensation for Cerebral Palsy (Investigation). Available from: http://www.sanka-hp.jcqhc.or.jp/documents/analysis/index.html [Accessed: June 01, 2022, in Japanese]

[12] Website of the Japan Obstetric Compensation for Cerebral Palsy (40th Steering Committee Paper). pp. 16-19. Available from: http://www.sanka-hp.jcqhc.or.jp/documents/committee/

obstetric_meeting40.pdf [Accessed: June 01, 2022, in Japanese]

[13] Website of the Japan Obstetric Compensation for Cerebral Palsy (41st Steering Committee Paper). pp. 14-16. Available from: http://www.sanka-hp.jcqhc.or.jp/documents/committee/obstetric_meeting41.pdf [Accessed: June 01, 2022, in Japanese]

[14] Website of the Japan Obstetric Compensation for Cerebral Palsy (41st Steering Committee Paper). pp. 15-21. Available from: http://www.sanka-hp.jcqhc.or.jp/documents/committee/obstetric_meeting43.pdf [Accessed: June 01, 2022, in Japanese]

[15] Website of the Japan Obstetric Compensation for Cerebral Palsy (Prevention: Overview): Available from: http://www.sanka-hp.jcqhc.or.jp/outline/prevention.html [Accessed: June 01, 2022, in Japanese]

[16] Website of the Japan Obstetric Compensation for Cerebral Palsy (Prevention: Annual Report). Available from: http://www.sanka-hp.jcqhc.or.jp/documents/prevention/report/ [Accessed: June 01, 2022, in Japanese]

[17] Website of the Japan Obstetric Compensation for Cerebral Palsy (Prevention: Educational Products). Available from: http://www.sanka-hp.jcqhc.or.jp/documents/prevention/proposition/ [Accessed: June 01, 2022, in Japanese]

[18] Website of the Japan Obstetric Compensation for Cerebral Palsy (Prevention: Textbook on CTG Interpretation). Available from: http://www.sanka-hp.jcqhc.or.jp/documents/english/pdf/Cardiotocograms_of_Cerebral_Palsy_Cases.pdf [Accessed: June 01, 2022, in Japanese]

[19] A Report on Expedition of Lawsuit-VI. Verification of Social Background Factors 4. Study on Conflict by Type." Issued by The Supreme Court of Japan. 2013. Available from: http://www.courts.go.jp/vcms_lf/20524011.pdf [Accessed: June 01, 2022, in Japanese]

[20] Website of the Japan Obstetric Compensation for Cerebral Palsy (1st Overhaul Committee Paper). Available from: http://www.sanka-hp.jcqhc.or.jp/documents/committee/pdf/kentou_meeting1_1.pdf; http://www.sanka-hp.jcqhc.or.jp/documents/committee/kentou_meeting1_2.pdf; http://www.sanka-hp.jcqhc.or.jp/documents/committee/kentou_meeting1_3.pdf [Accessed: June 01, 2022, in Japanese]

[21] Website of the Japan Obstetric Compensation for Cerebral Palsy (2nd Overhaul Committee Paper). Available from: http://www.sanka-hp.jcqhc.or.jp/documents/committee/pdf/kentou_meeting2_1.pdf [Accessed: June 01, 2022, in Japanese]

[22] Website of the Japan Obstetric Compensation for Cerebral Palsy (3rd Overhaul Committee Paper). Available from: http://www.sanka-hp.jcqhc.or.jp/documents/committee/pdf/kentou_meeting3_1.pdf [Accessed: June 01, 2022, in Japanese]

[23] Website of the Japan Obstetric Compensation for Cerebral Palsy (4th Overhaul Committee Paper). Available from: http://www.sanka-hp.jcqhc.or.jp/documents/committee/pdf/kentou_meeting4.pdf [Accessed: June 01, 2022, in Japanese]

[24] Website of the Japan Obstetric Compensation for Cerebral Palsy (Report on 2022 overhaul of the Japan Obstetric Compensation for Cerebral Palsy). Available from: http://www.sanka-hp.jcqhc.or.jp/documents/committee/pdf/minaoshinikansuruhoukokusho20201204.pdf [Accessed: June 01, 2022, in Japanese]